To Stanley
with v

Jonathan ...

Tinnitus

Tinnitus

Jonathan W. P. Hazell
MA, MB BChir, FRCS
Consultant Neuro-Otologist, Royal National Institute for the Deaf, London; Honorary Senior Lecturer in Neuro-Otology, University College, London; Honorary Consultant Neuro-Otologist, University College Hospital, London; Honorary Consultant in Audiological Medicine, Royal National Throat, Nose and Ear Hospital, London.

CHURCHILL LIVINGSTONE
EDINBURGH LONDON MELBOURNE AND NEW YORK 1987

CHURCHILL LIVINGSTONE
Medical Division of Longman Group UK Limited

Distributed in the United States of America by Churchill Livingstone Inc., 1560 Broadway, New York, N.Y. 10036, and by associated companies, branches and representatives throughout the world.

© Longman Group UK Limited 1987

All rights reserved. No part of this publication may be reproduced, stored in a retrieval system, or transmitted in any form or by any means, electronic, mechanical, photocopying, recording or otherwise, without the prior permission of the publishers (Churchill Livingstone, Robert Stevenson House, 1-3 Baxter's Place, Leith Walk, Edinburgh EH1 3AF).

First published 1987

ISBN 0-443-02156-2

British Library Cataloguing in Publication Data
Tinnitus.
　1. Tinnitus
　I. Hazell, Jonathan W. P.
　617.8　　RF293.8

Library of Congress Cataloging in Publication Data
Tinnitus
　Includes index.
　1. Tinnitus.　I. Hazell, Jonathan W. P.
[DNLM: 1. Tinnitus.　WV 272 T5912]
RF293.8.T554　1987　　617.8'86　　87-9311

Produced by Longman Singapore Publishers (Pte) Ltd.
Printed in Singapore.

Preface

It is only in the last five years that we have seen the appearance of books on the subject of tinnitus, as yet but a handful. This may be compared with the plethora of textbooks and lengthy publications on the subject of deafness and hearing impairment, in many of which the subject of tinnitus receives but a scant mention. Nevertheless, tinnitus has been shown to be at least as common as hearing impairment and arguably as much a handicap. Those unfortunate enough to have lost all their hearing and to suffer from tinnitus almost always complain that the problem of communication is dwarfed by the difficulties of living with an incessant cacophony of noise inside their head from which there is not a moment's relief. However, over a quarter of tinnitus sufferers will not experience any communication difficulties, and until recently would have had nowhere to go to find sympathy and understanding about their complaint. It is hard for even the most kindly physician to offer more than a short homily about a condition which he does not understand and cannot treat.

In recent years, the interest in tinnitus has increased dramatically in the scientific community. Now that auditory physiologists have turned their minds to tackling the problem of what tinnitus really is and how it is generated, this symptom may be seen at last as a real entity which demands as much of our time and energy as the problems of hearing impairment; it is at least as common. Just as the presentation of different kinds of hearing loss can give us insight into the pathological processes involved, so tinnitus must be telling us something about the processes at work in the auditory system. Measurements of this elusive and often variable symptom do not at present afford us a great deal of scientific insight into the working of the ear, but a dismissive attitude to this symptom in the past has, I believe, led to a loss of much useful clinical information. There are still a great many unanswered questions about tinnitus. Not the least of these is why almost a third of those with severe hearing impairment have no tinnitus whatever. It is my wish that this volume should help to promote interest in the problem of tinnitus among workers in this field, to increase our understanding of the mechanisms involved, and to avoid that familiar situation where the sufferer from tinnitus is told by his medical adviser that there is nothing to be done, and that he must 'learn to live with it'.

London, 1987   J. W. P. H.

Acknowledgements

This book belongs to my co-authors, all of whom are well-known for their involvement in the field of tinnitus. I cannot thank them enough for their eager and instant agreement to contribute to this volume and their prompt delivery. (Other prospective editors please note!)

The stimulus for this book and the help I have received in its production comes from sources too numerous to mention. I am deeply grateful to the Royal National Institute for the Deaf, London, who since 1974 have funded the research programme on tinnitus, and without whose continued support and encouragement nothing would have been achieved. Mike Martin, OBE, who first took me under his wing, has been a constant source of ideas and provided much technical support. Successive research assistants Sue Meadows (née Wood), Huw Cooper and Leah Meerton have all contributed to the research programme and thus ultimately to this book. Pat Garrett, our research secretary, has manipulated our word processor with consummate skill and has organized the illustrations and collation of the manuscript. I am extremely grateful to her. Mary Plackett and her staff in the RNID library have provided an invaluable service in tracking down references, and Helen Bacon has checked each one in the final text, with meticulous care.

I am particularly grateful for the advice and help received from Harald Feldmann, whose classical paper on homolateral and contralateral masking of tinnitus made me realize in the early days that this was a subject that could be researched. Jack Vernon and the pioneering work of the Kresge Institute in Portland, Oregon, USA, have helped and considerably influenced the development of our own clinical services and ideas about masking techniques. In the UK the influence of Jack Ashley, ChB, MP, has done much to establish the status of tinnitus as a serious subject for research and clinical support. I am deeply grateful for his personal interest in the research programme and in the production of this volume. He was the catalyst in the Ciba Foundation Symposium No. 85 on tinnitus which was held in London in 1981 and which resulted in probably the first modern book on the subject of tinnitus and from which numerous references have been taken in these chapters. He was the driving force behind the establishment of the British Tinnitus Association, which has given such valuable support to tinnitus sufferers all over the country. I would like to thank my colleagues at University College Hospital, London, and especially Graham Fraser for his constant support and good advice.

I am indebted to all those in the UCH tinnitus clinic, for their unfailing support throughout our clinical trials (and tribulations!) and, in particular, Sheila McDonald and Jane Butler for their faultless audiometry. Finally, I must thank all those lay workers in the field of tinnitus, members of the British Tinnitus Association and others, many of whom suffer from tinnitus themselves, who have given support, raised funds and been very largely responsible for the scientific advances that have been made in this subject by their ceaseless insistence that something can be done.

Contributors

Karen I. Berliner PhD
Director of Clinical Research, House Ear Institute, Los Angeles, CA 90057, USA; Adjunct Assistant Professor of Psychiatry and the Behavioral Sciences, University of Southern California School of Medicine, USA.

James K. Cunningham PhD
Research Methodologist, House Ear Institute, Los Angeles, California, USA.

Ronald J. Goodey BMedSc, MBChB, FRACS
Clinical Lecturer in Charge of Otolaryngology, Auckland University School of Medicine; Visiting Otolaryngologist, Greenlane Hospital, Auckland 3, New Zealand.

John M. Graham MA, BM, BCh, FRCS (Eng), FRCS (Ed)
Consultant ENT Surgeon, University College Hospital, London, UK.

Richard S. Hallam BA, MSc, PhD, DipPsychol
Principal Clinical Psychologist (Bloomsbury Health Authority); Senior Lecturer in Psychology, The Middlesex Hospital Medical School, London, UK.

Jonathan W. P. Hazell MA, MBBChir, FRCS
Consultant Neuro-Otologist to the Royal National Institute for the Deaf, London; Honorary Senior Lecturer in Neuro-Otology, University College, London; Honorary Consultant Neuro-Otologist, University College Hospital, London; Honorary Consultant in Audiological Medicine, Royal National Throat, Nose and Ear Hospital, London, UK.

MRC Institute of Hearing Research, University Park, Nottingham, UK. The chapter was prepared by Dr R. A. Coles, Assistant Director and Coordinator of Clinical Studies, in collaboration with Dr A. C. Davis and Professor M. P. Haggard.

S. Dai G. Stephens BSc, MPhil, MRCP
Physician in Charge, Welsh Hearing Institute, University Hospital of Wales, Cardiff, UK.

Jack Vernon PhD
Professor of Otolaryngology, Oregon Health Sciences University; Director, Oregon Health Sciences Hearing Research Center, Portland, Oregon, USA.

J. Patrick Wilson BSc, PhD
Senior Research Fellow, Department of Communication and Neuroscience, University of Keele, UK.

Contents

1. Historical aspects of tinnitus 1
   S. D. G. Stephens
2. Theory of tinnitus generation 20
   J. P. Wilson
3. Epidemiology of tinnitus in adults 46
   MRC Institute of Hearing Research, UK
4. Assessment of the tinnitus patient 71
   J. Vernon
5. Tinnitus masking therapy 96
   J. W. P. Hazell
6. Tinnitus suppression in cochlear implantation 118
   K. I. Berliner and J. K. Cunningham
7. Tinnitus in hearing-impaired children 131
   J. M. Graham
8. Surgical management of the tinnitus patient 144
   J. W. P. Hazell
9. Psychological approaches to the evaluation and management of tinnitus distress 156
   R. S. Hallam
10. Drug therapy in tinnitus 176
    R. J. Goodey
11. Guidelines for the management of tinnitus 195
    J. W. P. Hazell

    Index 197

1
S. D. G. Stephens

Historical aspects of tinnitus

The English word 'tinnitus' is dated by the Oxford English Dictionary to 1963 when, in the second edition of Blanchard's Physicians' Dictionary, *Tinnitus aurium* was defined as 'a certain buzzing or tingling in the ears'. It is derived from the Latin *tinnire*, to ring.

Prior to that time, for example, the section on tinnitus in the Middle English version of Gilbertus Anglicus (Getz 1981) is entitled 'Ringing in the ears' and starts: 'Ringing in a mannes eris, or oþere noise liche blowing of hornes, commeþ in diuerse maneris: oþerwhiles, of a grete wyndi mater þat is in þe eere and moveþ vp and dovun and al abouten withinforpe and may not oute for his boistesnes, and þerfore þer is a contynuel ringing and noyse in þe eeres.'

In the early 17th century, Francis Bacon in his 'Sylva Sylvarum' (1627) talks merely about 'a loud ringing (not an ordinary singing and hissing but far louder and differing)' following exposure to an explosion. Even in the English translation of Du Verney's 'Traité de l'organ de l'ouie' published in London in 1737, there is a discussion of various types of noises associated with ear disease, but the word 'tinnitus' is not used.

In the French language, unlike English, a number of different words have been used for tinnitus. These include 'bourdonnements', 'tintements', 'tintouins', 'acouphènes' and 'sifflements', and the origins of these are discussed by Guerrier & Mounier-Kuhn (1980). However, even these authors consider that the term 'bourdonnements', one of the relative newcomers, dating only from the 17th century, has largely superseded the others.

This chapter, however, will be concerned with the historical development of ideas of the origins of tinnitus and its treatment. Elsewhere I have discussed the history of the treatment of tinnitus and its management in the context of the facilitation of the habituation process (Stephens 1984, 1985). The habituation model of tinnitus is discussed elsewhere in this book by Hallam (see Ch. 9). Within this presentation I shall consider the treatments, particularly in the context of the current views of the cause or causes of the symptom.

THE EARLIEST IDEAS

Little has been written of 'primitive' tribal medical views of tinnitus. Politzer (1907) documents information from Bartel's (1893) work on 'The medicine of primitive tribes' referring particularly to the views of the Annamites of Eastern India. They believed that the ear is inhabited by a small animal whose function is to protect the ear. If it engages in a fight with similar animals or is disturbed by a foreign body, tinnitus ensues. Diseases of the ear causing such problems were treated by fumigation with the burning of skins of non-poisonous snakes.

Such a treatment may seem rational, given the hypothesis of the cause of the symptom, and undoubtedly similar concepts occurred among many of our ancestors at a time when such information was not documented.

The earliest surviving medical documentation comes in papyruses of ancient Egypt and the clay tablets of the Babylonian/Assyrian culture. Among the early Egyptian papyruses which have survived and which refer to ear disease, the Ebers papyrus is probably the best known, dealing with medical illnesses and their treatment. Although this papyrus dates back to the 16th century BC, it is generally considered (e.g. Kamal 1968) to be a copy of early papyruses from as early as 2500 BC, the time of the construction of the great pyramids. While tinnitus is not explicitly mentioned in the Ebers papyrus, it is often thought that one section (no. 678) refers to tinnitus – 'Treatment for a bewitched ear – balanites oil 1 portion, frankincense 1 portion, (Sekhopf?) 1 portion – infused into the ear'. Such infusions were common in the treatment of ear disease in ancient Egypt, perhaps stemming from the fact that much of it was caused by otitis media, as indicated by the descriptions in the papyruses and by modern studies on the skulls of mummies.

The Edwin Smith papyrus deals primarily with the treatment of injuries, including those to the ear, and the Berlin papyrus presents treatments similar to those found in the Ebers documentation (Leca 1971). However, Leca also refers to the 'Ostracon médical du Louvre, No. 3235' in which fumigation of the ears with various exotic substances is used.

In a late papyrus from Crocodilopolis, parts of which are thought to date back to the 6th century BC (Reymond 1976), treatment for 'humming in the ears' is specifically mentioned. This entailed the introduction of a variety of herbs, oils and salt to the external ear via a hollow reed stalk. Some of these treatments must have been effective, even if only in reassuring the patient and facilitating the habituation process, judging by the number of votive ears which have been found in the temples of Thebes and Memphis.

Unlike the Egyptians, the Assyrians preserved their medical documentation on clay tablets. Thanks to the work of Campbell Thompson (1931) we have fairly extensive documentation of the views of that time on the causes, types and treatment of tinnitus. These date back at least to the seventh century BC. Following on the Egyptian theme of the ears being bewitched, the Assyrians make repeated statements along the lines of: 'if the hand of a ghost seizes on a man and his ears sing . . .'. In addition there is one reference which appears to be to the tinnitus interfering with the individual's hearing: 'if a man's right ear speaks, a bar (shutting) him . . .'. I have discussed elsewhere (Stephens 1984) the three types of tinnitus alluded to in these tablets, the 'singing' (? ringing tinnitus), 'whispering' (? hissing) and 'speaking' (?? auditory hallucinations) and the fact that the last two may be referred to specifically as left and right and sometimes be treated with purging medications. In fact, among the references to the treatment of tinnitus in this text, while there are 19 to 'ears' singing, there is only one for the right ear only and one for the left ear only, in each case for the ear 'whispering' or 'speaking'.

The 'whispering' is treated in both cases with an incantation, accompanied in the case of the left ear by the use of turmeric and the insertion into the external ear of wool sprinkled ritually three times with an unknown substance. In the case of the ears 'speaking', purging food over the magical period of seven days is prescribed, mustard in beer for the right ear, dates and unknown other substances for the left.

Singing in the ears was not treated by purging, but rather by the recitation of incantations, often together with wool impregnated with various oils inserted into the external ear or with various similar substances inserted directly into the external canal, sometimes through a bronze tube. In yet other cases, fumigations with burning aromatic substances are recommended. The incantations vary from brief calls to the ghost to leave the person, to long verses such as:

Oh thou that spieth,
Oh thou that spieth,
Oh thou that pursueth,
Whatever its name,
Though on earth art seed of the heavens,
Unto his form as of heaven,
Come not nigh:
Like a mountain thou restrainest,
His form thou hast troubled . . .
O ye four devils of the roads,
O ye four devils of the ways . . .
Get ye to your four quarters . . .
May Ninurta, lord of the sword,
Turn you back.
O by heaven be ye exorcised,
By earth be ye exorcised!

Ninurta has been described as 'champion of the celestial gods' and 'the strong one who destroys the wicked and the enemy'. His attribute was a kind of club flanked by two S shaped snakes (Guirand 1959). A similar incantation, but in that case calling on Ea god of the physicians and god of knowledge for similar help, has been referred to in Stephens (1984).

Overall, it may be seen that the treatment is again well in keeping with concepts of the causation of the tinnitus and aimed at soothing the patient, reassuring him that something meaningful could be done. This in turn would facilitate the process of habituation to the tinnitus.

GRAECO-ROMAN MEDICINE

Many of the concepts in medicine in this period were related to Empedocles' (490–430 BC) theory of the humours. Dysbalance of these humours could lead to a variety of symptoms, one of which was tinnitus. In parallel with this humoral theory was a more practical and pragmatic approach based on empirical observations. Little, however, has survived from a theoretical point of view outlining the details of contemporary views on tinnitus. Even among the copious writings of the Hippocratic Corpus, there is little. Tinnitus is explained as a perception of pulsation in the cranial blood vessels (Politzer 1907) and as a cause of headaches. Such headaches should not be treated by purging (Littré 1984) as this treatment may prevent spontaneous recovery of the symptom. Tinnitus was commonly described as occurring during fevers, following loss of blood, and at the beginning of menstruation.

In the first century AD, Celsus published a compendium of treatments under the title of 'De medicina'. He is thought not to have been a physician, but rather a private gentleman of a noble family who collected these for practical purposes. Book VI, section VII deals with ear disease and part 8 of this with tinnitus. It starts: 'Aliud viti genus est, ubi aures intra se ipsas onant; atque hoc quoque fit, ne externum sonum accipiant. (Another type of lesion is that in which the ears produce a ringing sound within them; and this also prevents them from perceiving external sounds.)' (Spencer 1938).

Such tinnitus was divided into that which is least serious when caused by a cold in the head, worse when related to diseases or prolonged pains in the head, and worst when it indicated the onset of serious illness, in particular epilepsy. Tinnitus related to colds was cleared by aural toilet and Valsalva's manoeuvre, being apparently associated with a perforated tympanic membrane. Tinnitus related to disease or pain in the head should be treated by exercise, massage, effusion and gargling with dieting. Various juices and oils might be introduced into the external ear, sometimes mixed up into a salve. If there was no such obvious cause for the tinnitus, and it had sinister implications, Celsus recommended similar oils to be applied to the external ear, dieting and abstinence from the consumption of wine. This is one of the earliest reports of a relationship between alcohol and tinnitus.

Galen (130–200 AD) was both a collector of others' work and an original thinker himself. While Hippocrates may be regarded in many ways as the father of Greek medicine, Galen, with his voluminous writings, had most influence on medical practice until at least the Renaissance. He advocated a variety of treatments for tinnitus, mainly entailing the introduction of liquid and semifluid substances into the external ear. While some of these may well have had useful soothing effects, he still included certain quasi-magical treatments, more generally associated with Pliny, such as the instillation of cockroaches ground up in rose oil to the external ear for the treatment of tinnitus associated with pain (Kuhn 1965). He did, however, in other cases of tinnitus, recommend dulling the senses with mandrake or opium.

BYZANTINE, ARABIC AND MEDIAEVAL MEDICINE

From a theoretical point of view, Galen supported Aristotle's (384-322 BC) view of there being implanted air within the ear. This view was elaborated by Alexander of Tralles (525-605 AD) with regard to tinnitus, arguing as he did that it was caused by the air being dense and expanding with no outlet. This was a view seized upon more than a millenium later by Jean Riolan the Younger (1580-1657) who advocated trepanning the mastoid to let such air escape, as a means of treating the tinnitus. This idea of tinnitus being caused by an 'accumulation' of 'vapours' within the ear recurred throughout mediaeval and later times. Mesue (d. 1015) felt that such vapours might be accumulated in the head and Bernard de Gordon (1305) described these vapours as causing violent vibrations in the inner part of the ear. The subjective impressions differed according to the quality of the sound produced by the vapours, being a murmuring, rushing, tingling, bubbling, etc. The treatments were somewhat traditional (Politzer 1907).

As discussed elsewhere (Stephens 1984), other classifications and treatments of tinnitus throughout mediaeval times largely follow on from the approach of Celsus. Thus Paul of Aegina (625–690 AD) divided tinnitus into that occurring during fevers, that due to 'thick and viscid humours, and the chronic noises and hissing sounds (Adams 1844). Avicenna (980–1036) added those 'caused by excitement of the senses' to this classification, and Gilbertus Anglicus, among others, included tinnitus related to 'feebleness of the ears'. The treatments for these all followed the general lines of oily or other liquid or emulsified substances administered to the external ear, accompanied in certain cases by various forms of mild purging. In some writings, the fumigation of the ears is included, either as a treatment in itself, or as a prelude to direct application of other substances to the external ear canal, as described by Guy de Chauliac (1300–1370) (see Ogden 1971).

The types of substances administered directly to the external ear recur through most of the mediaeval times and similar, or at least overlapping, ranges of substances have been used for various types of aural symptoms such as otalgia, hearing loss and otorrhoea, in addition to tinnitus. These have been discussed by Opsomer-Halleux (1981).

In addition to this mainstream continuation of classical approaches, a number of incidental and often important findings about tinnitus and its management were noted and recorded by various mediaeval physicians. Thus, Alisaundre (? Alexander of Tralles 525–605 AD) is described by Guy de Chauliac as relating that tinnitus sufferers obtain relief 'to walke in sondry places'. Guy de Chauliac goes on to report Avicenna as saying: 'To crye and to excite him with crying voice is profitable' (Ogden 1971). This idea of obtaining relief by external noises either by masking, distraction or subsequent suppression of the tinnitus is also articulated by Pseudo Aristotle from the School of Salerno (ca. 13th century) who asks in the 'Problemata': 'Why is it that buzzing in the ears ceases if one makes a sound? Is it because a greater sound drives out the less?' (Forster 1927).

At the same time, specific causes of tinnitus were being described. Avicenna referred to tinnitus being caused by specific remedies 'leading to retention of humours and winds in certain parts of the brain' (Avicenna 1964). Wright (1985) has shown that Avicenna described an ototoxic effect of mercury inhalations on hearing ability, so that it is possible that here he could also have been referring to the effects of this therapy.

Valescus of Tranta (1418) reported tinnitus caused by a blow to the head. He also mentioned that following blows to the ears as a punishment for boys' misbehaviour, tinnitus and hearing loss occurred quite commonly (Politzer 1907).

THE RENAISSANCE TO THE 19th CENTURY

These lines of development continued throughout this time. Francis Bacon (1560-1626) in 'Sylva Sylvarum' (1627) refers to the temporary tinnitus experienced after an explosion. 'A very great sound, near hand, hath strucken many deaf; and at the instant they have found, as it were, the breaking of a skin of parchment in their ear: and myself standing near the one that lured loud and shrill, had suddenly an offence as if somewhat had broken or been dislocated in my ear; and immediately after a loud ringing (not an ordinary singing or hissing, but far louder and differing) so as I feared some deafness. But after some half quarter of an hour, it vanished'. Paracelsus (1491–1541), about a century earlier, had reported that tinnitus was often due to exposure to loud noises.

Following the siege of Naples after Columbus' return from the Americas, syphilis spread rapidly through Europe. Fallopius, in his 'De morbo gallico (About the French disease)' (1563) commented that tinnitus due to syphilis was incurable. Whether he considered that this was due to the syphilis *per se* or to its treatment with mercury or to both was uncertain.

Others expressed the view that tinnitus was caused by the air trapped within the ear, and Johannes Fernelius (1497–1558) had described different types of tinnitus as being attributable to differential rates of escape of this air (Politzer 1907). It seems likely that the approaches to treating the tinnitus by the application of suction to the ear, which date back to John of Gaddesden (1280?–1361), depend on the same theory. Instruments were not available at the time to enable the physician to examine the tympanic membrane.

The 17th century saw an increase in interest in tinnitus, and dissertations devoted to the topic began to be published. A number of these, based in part on Politzer's bibliography (1907) and in part on the author's collection, are listed in Table 1.1. It is of note that Hartmann's dissertation (1669) was performed under the supervision of Schenck (1619–1671), whose dissertation had been published two years earlier. Bolland's (1694) was under the supervision of Krause (1642-1718), although in this case there was a gap of 13 years between the two publications.

Table 1.1 Dissertations on Tinnitus published in the 17th and 18th Centuries

Zeidler (1630) Dissertationem de aurium tinnitu. Leipzig.
Johann Theodor Schenck (1667) Dissertationem de tinnitu aruium. Jena.
Martinus Hartmann (1669) Dissertationem inauguralem medicam de tinnitu aurium. Jena.
Rudolfus Guilielmus Crausius (Rudolf Wilhelm Krause) (1681). Dissertationem de tinnitu aurium. Jena.
Johannes Jonas Bolland (1694) Disputatio inauguralis medica de tinnitu aurium. Jena.
Helbich (1699) Dissertationem de sonitu et tinnitu aurium. Altdorf.
Jakob Finckenau (1706) Dissertationem de tinnitu aurium. Konigsberg.
Johannis Fr. Cartheuser (1770) Dissertationem de susurratione et tinnitus aurium. Frankfurt.
J H Schedel (1784) Dissertationem de tinnitu aurium. Duisburg.
Johannis Gottlieb Liedenfrost (1787) Dissertationem de tinnitu aurium. Duisburg.

The title pages of the dissertations by Hartmann and by Bolland are shown in Figures 1.1 and 1.2. These two are largely concerned with a reiteration of aetiological and therapeutic views dating back to classical times. The contents of the two overlap very considerably. It is interesting to note that Hartmann (1669) included vascular pulsation as a common cause of tinnitus. Among the less common causes he included the supernatural, a hereditary disposition to the condition and depression. He reported that syphilis was a rare cause of tinnitus and that eunuchs were immune from the symptom! Bolland (1694) repeated much of the contents of Hartmann's dissertation in his own, but advocated a holistic approach to the management of tinnitus with moderation in behaviour and diet, avoiding extremes of cold and heat, neither sleeping nor staying awake in excess, and refraining from too much sexual exertion.

In the middle of the 17th century, Jean Riolan the younger (1580–1657) had introduced the concept of trepanning the mastoid to allow the air which was rushing around inside it (causing the tinnitus) to escape (1649). This was based on the concepts discussed earlier and reiterated in the two dissertations. However, this approach later became discredited following the deaths of one or two eminent individuals on whom it was later practised (Politzer 1907).

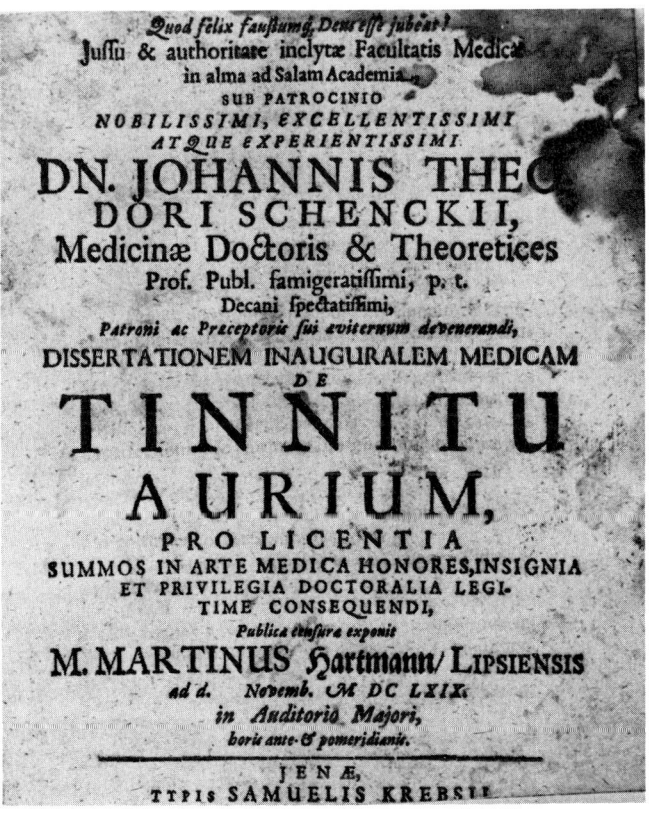

Fig. 1.1 Title page of Hartmann (1669).

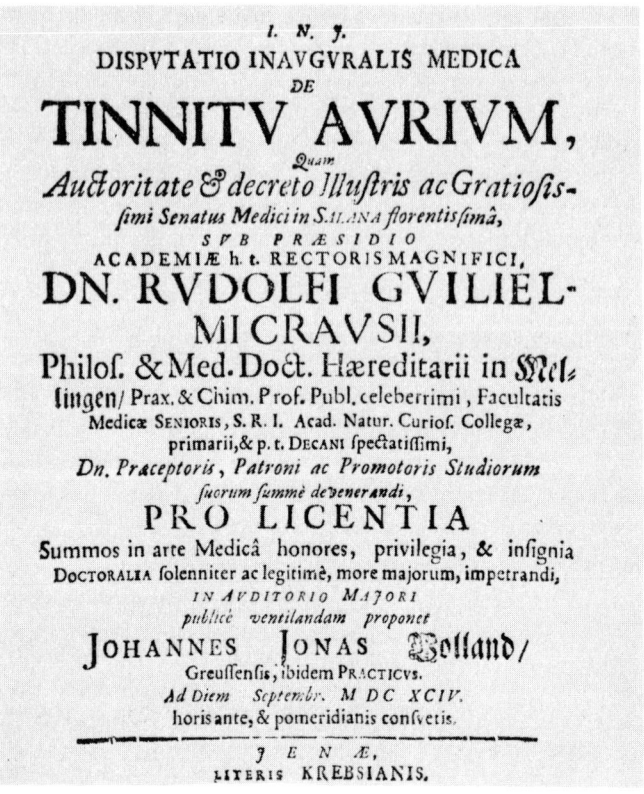

Fig. 1.2 Title page of Bolland (1694).

The publication of Du Verney's (1648-1730) 'Traité de l'organ de l'ouie' in 1683 constituted an important milestone in otology, representing as it did, the first major textbook on the subject. As such, it was translated from the original French into Latin, English, German and Dutch with 12 editions being published between 1683 and 1750 (Asherson 1979). Within this text, ten pages (in the English edition of 1737) were devoted to tinnitus. Du Verney discarded the view of tinnitus being caused by air internus rushing round and round, and attributed it rather to vibrations within the ear on one hand and hyperexcitability within the nerves on the other. The latter was attributed to brain disease and the former to diseases of the ear. These last may arise in various parts of the ear and include arterial pulsations. He also illustrated how external ear obstructions could cause tinnitus by drawing parallels with the sounds heard when the external meatus is occluded by the hand. Finally, he argued that any treatment should be aimed at the underlying ear or brain disease rather than at the symptom *per se*.

Johann Jakob Wepfer's (1620–1695) views (1727) were somewhat less sophisticated but in general overall agreement, and were published only posthumously. One interesting theory which he resurrected was that of suppressing the tinnitus with loud noises. In one case he described his management as follows: '... prope aurum duos lapillos crebrius allisit, ut sonitus percussorum lapillorum obstaculum removeret'.*

Following the development of Eustachian catheterization by Giot and others in the early 18th century various physicians focused on Eustachian tube obstruction as a cause of tinnitus. Thus Cartheuser (1770) attributed whistling tinnitus to a defect of the Eustachian tube and Leschevin (1732–1788) in 1776 extended this view, stating that the Eustachian obstruction led to rarefaction of the air within the middle ear, so causing the symptom.

The use of static electricity in therapy dates back to 1749 and was widely applied by the 1770s (Garrison 1929). It was thus not surprising that it should be used in ear disease in general and in tinnitus in particular. In 1768 George Daniel Wibel in his dissertation 'Casum aegroti auditu difficili' reported 'Tandem nostra praecipue aevo Electicitatis vis in audiendi difficultate & tinnitu aurium sese commendavit egregie, quod pluribus exemplis probatur'†—indicating encouraging initial results with the technique. Recently, Feldmann (1984) has shown that almost immediately after Volta devised his famous Voltaic pile (1799) as a source of steady-state electricity (see Volta 1800), this was applied by Grapengiesser (1801) in the treatment of tinnitus. He used a variety of different electrode configurations including one electrode to be placed at the opening of the Eustachian tube. Feldmann reports that cathodal stimulation was more effective than positive polarity stimulation, although the later work in the 19th century (Bremner 1868) sugggested that the converse was true. It is interesting to note that about the same time as Grapengiesser was applying Volta's pile to the treatment of tinnitus, Erasmus Darwin (1731–1802) was using it to treat vertigo, in this case applying electrodes to the patient's temple (King-Hele 1981).

TINNITUS IN THE 19th CENTURY

My consideration of this period in the treatment of tinnitus will be restricted largely to two publications: Itard's 'Traité des maladies de l'oreille et de l'audition' published in 1821, and MacNaughton-Jones' 'Subjective noises in the head and ears', published in 1891. Itard's work represents the culmination of the observational approach to medicine developed by the Parisian school, and MacNaughton-Jones brings together much of the experience and knowledge accumulated through the century.

Jean Marie Gaspard Itard (1775–1838) is best known for his work with the prelingually deaf, and particularly for his efforts to teach speech to the wild boy of Aveyron (Lane 1976). His 'Traité des maladies die l'oreille et de l'audition' (Fig. 1.3) published in two volumes in 1821 was an important milestone in the management of ear disease, including also a description of one of the earliest mechanical audiometers (Stephens 1981), together with a variety of non-electrical hearing aids/ear trumpets (Stephens & Goodwin 1984). Among the more medical parts of the book, Itard devotes 26 pages of the second volume to tinnitus, including a classification, medical

---

* He banged two pebbles together next to his ear, so that the sound made by these stones would solve his problem.
† Finally the strength of static electricity was highly recommended for hearing problems and tinnitus, as may be shown by many examples.

Fig. 1.3 Title page of Itard (1821), Vol. 2.

treatments and the earliest extensive discussion of tinnitus masking. Tinnitus is described as one of the auditory 'deprivations' together with a variety of auditory distortions.

He started by rejecting the earlier terminology based on different names for tinnitus such as 'bruissement, murmure, sifflement, bombement, tintement etc.' and concentrated rather on a functional classification. He divided the tinnitus into three groups: true tinnitus (le bourdonnement vrai), false tinnitus (le bourdonnement faux) and fantastic tinnitus (le bourdonnement fantastique). The last, which he described as rare, he considered to be a symptom of a psychological disorder (aliénation mentale) and should be treated by treating the underlying psychological condition.

True tinnitus he felt to have an acoustical basis, such as the pulsation of arteries, a mechanical obstruction or general vasodilation. He felt, incorrectly, that if air arriving at the ear had to pass narrow obstructions, this in itself could cause tinnitus, drawing on the analogy of air escaping from a pipe. He considered false tinnitus, which he described as being much more common, to be generally due to damage to the cochlear nerve. Ideopathic false tinnitus generally occurred in ears which had earlier been exposed to acoustic trauma or noise trauma. Symptomatic false tinnitus, in which the tinnitus is one of a variety of psychosomatic symptoms, occurred particularly in office workers, hypochondriacs and hysterical women. It could also occur in patients with serious medical conditions such as severe haemorrhages and menorrhagia.

He commented on the severe psychological effects which tinnitus may have on the sufferers, leading them to seek all sorts of bizarre and painful treatments. Some of his own treatments, however, fall in this category, particularly for true tinnitus caused by 'un afflux trop considérable du sang vers la tête'. These should be treated by irritant footbaths, applications of leeches to the legs or bleeding, in severe cases even of the jugular vein. These treatments should be accompanied by cold douches to the head. He was obliged to admit, however, that often even such extreme treatments only had a temporary effect.

Itard suggested that false tinnitus should be treated by ether applied directly to the external auditory canal, but again admitted that such treatment was often unsuccessful. Treatment then should be directed towards relieving the effects of the tinnitus on the patient, the most important of which, he considered, was sleep disturbance. He described the production of various masking noises in the patient's bedroom to relieve this, the noise matching the tinnitus.

'Ainsi, celui que produit un feu de cheminée bein actif, soulage considerablement l'incommodité de ces bourdonnements sourds qui simulent le murmure lointain des vents et d'une rivière debordée. Le même moyen peut s'adapter encore au sifflement de l'oreille, en aliment le feu avec du bois vert ou légèrement mouillé. Lorsque le tintement imite le son des cloches, on le couvre aisément, pourvu qu'il ne soit pas très-fort, par le résonnement que produit un grand bassin de cuivre dans lequel tombe de haut un filet d'eau fourni par un vase d'égal capacité, percé a son fond d'une très petite ouverture. Dans les cas enfin ou l'oreille est fatiguée par un bruit semblable a celui d'un rouage en mouvement, on peut placer au chevet du lit quelque mécanique bruyante, mise en jeu par le débandement lent d'un ressort, et adapté à un jeu d'orgue ou à quelque pendule grossière, dont on accelere le mouvement en otant le balancier' (Itard 1821).*

---

* Thus, producing a roaring fire in the grate considerably relieves the disturbance resulting from tinnitus which sounds like the distant murmuring of wind and a river in flood. The same approach can be adopted with whistling tinnitus, by putting green or slightly damp wood on the fire. When the tinnitus is like the sound of bells, as long as it is not too loud, it may be masked by the resonance of a large copper bowl into which falls a trickle of water from a vase of the same capacity, with a tiny hole pierced in its base. Finally in the case of tinnitus resembling the sound of a set of wheels turning, one can place alongside the bed a noisy spring-driven motor, adapted to a mechanical organ, or a large watch, of which the movements are speeded up by removal of the regulator.

Here we have the first practical description of a comprehensive approach to tinnitus masking, and Itard went on to say that despite the fact that such noises are louder than the patient's tinnitus, they do in fact help him to sleep profoundly. Among the case histories that he included following this, he described a lady who had severe tinnitus following psychological trauma from which she obtained relief only by living for several months in a water mill.

The eminent physiologist Johannes Müller (1801–1858) discussed the mechanism of tinnitus in his 'Handbuch der Physiologie des Menschen' (1834–40). He considered that subjective noises were due to overstimulation of the auditory nerve accompanying cerebral diseases, neural weakness or diseases of the auditory nerve itself. Tinnitus of the type referred to by Itard as 'true tinnitus', was due to aneurysmal dilatation of vessels, crackling sounds from the middle ear muscles, or buzzing from the contraction of the palatine muscles (Politzer 1907).

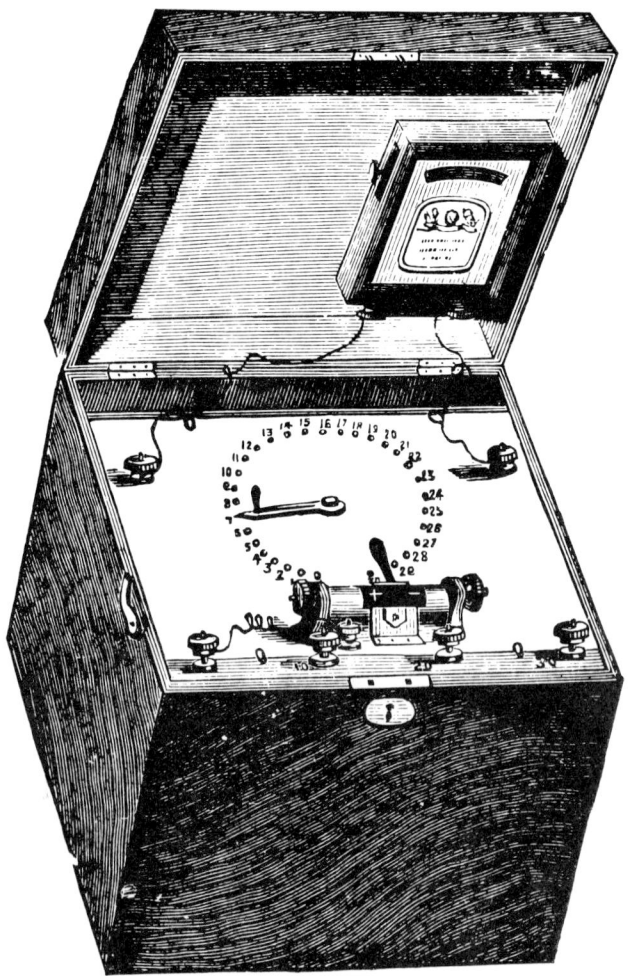

Fig. 1.4 Galvanic battery used by MacNaughton Jones (1891).

Through most of the remainder of the 19th century, despite major progress in other aspects of medicine, there was little development in the treatment of tinnitus. Certain techniques became more sophisticated, ineffective drugs were replaced by more modern ineffective drugs and many otological textbooks completely ignored the symptom, or at best devoted a paltry paragraph or two to it. William Wilde (1853) extolled the virtue of myringotomy on the one hand and leeches on the other. He was, however, honest enough to admit 'it is certainly one of the most distressing as well as one of the most frequent symptoms attendant upon afflictions of the organs of hearing, but its cause is very obscure and difficult to comprehend, and its removal still more difficult to achieve' (Wilde 1853).

Brenner (1868) developed a more sophisticated approach to the electrical suppression of tinnitus using the more advanced batteries, commutators, and rheostats which had become available by that time. Figure 1.4 shows such an electricity source used by MacNaughton Jones and illustrated in his book on tinnitus (1891). The 'indifferent' electrode (a metal plate) was placed on the back of the neck, and the active electrode, a sponge, placed to occlude the external meatus completely. MacNaughton Jones was not convinced of the efficacy of this treatment, commenting (pp. 131-132) 'in cases of which it has done good I have always been in doubt if the benefit was not as much derived from other treatment accompanying its use as from the galvanism alone'.

Despite this approach to more 'orthodox' galvanism, MacNaughton-Jones used a complex electrical stimulation technique when he thought that the tinnitus was related to a lack of tone in the muscles of the Eustachian tube. For this he advocated faradization of the muscles, using a faradic battery (Fig. 1.5a) the current from which was taken to an electrode on a Eustachian catheter (Fig. 1.5b) with a second sponge electrode in the external meatus attached to an aural speculum (Fig. 1.5c). However, even with this exotic approach, he is forced to admit 'it has often disappointed me'. Returning to the more general aspects, MacNaughton-Jones first divided tinnitus into the nine classes below.

1. Impulses arising from irritation of the central nervous system
2. Impulses arising from irritation of the auditory nerve
3. Impulses arising from the peripheral ends of the auditory nerve due to:
    a. Changes in labyrinthine pressure
    b. Vascular changes
    c. Morbid nerve conditions
    d. Rheumatic, gouty or syphilitic states
    e. Reflected systemic disease
4. Irritations from the intratympanic muscles
5. Irritations transmitted by altered air equilibration in the tympanic cavity
6. Irritations due to disease in the middle ear and labyrinth
7. Irritations arising in the external ear
8. True aural hallucinations:
    a. Arising in the brain when the auditory system is healthy
    b. Secondary to objective changes in the aural apparatus
9. Therapeutic causes of tinnitus aurium.

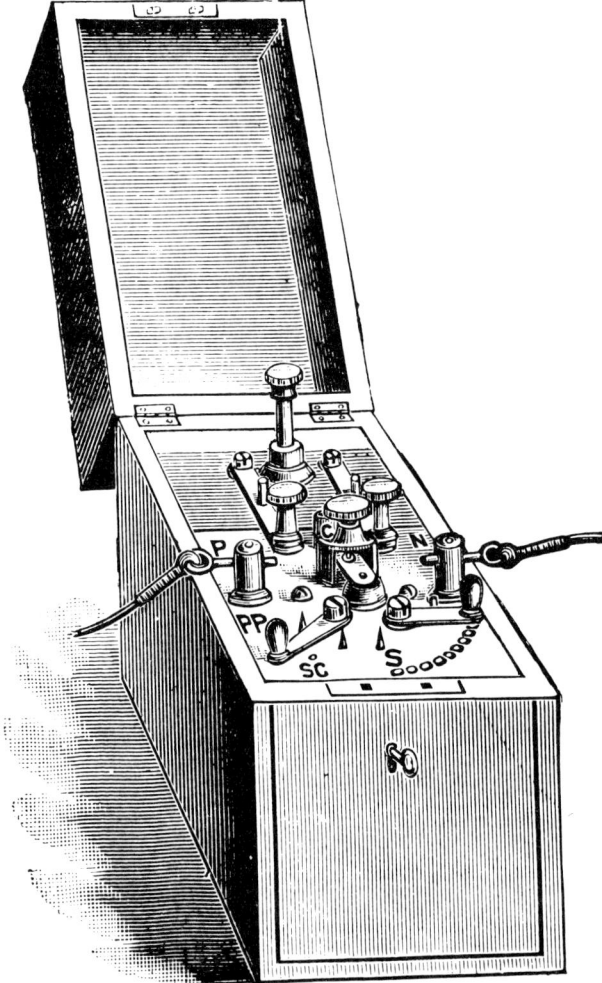

Fig. 1.5a Faradic battery.

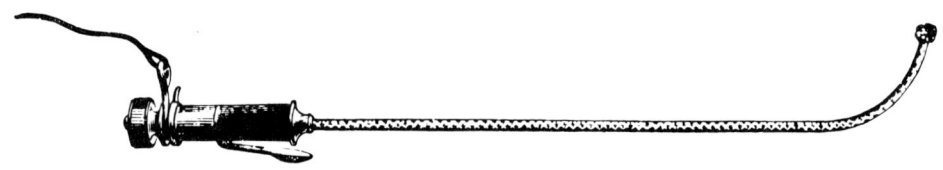

Fig. 1.5b Eustachian tube electrode.

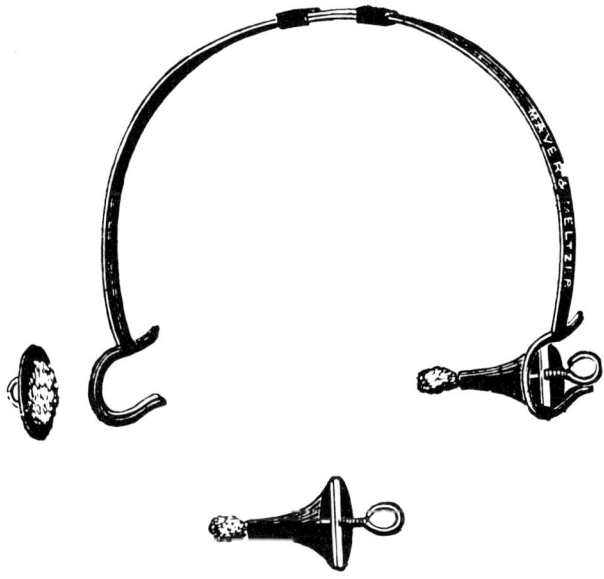

Fig. 1.5c External ear electrode. (Reproduced with permission from MacNaughton Jones 1891.)

As I have indicated elsewhere (Stephens 1984) many of the drugs listed under Class 9 are also advocated elsewhere in his publication for the treatment of tinnitus, a picture which had not changed 90 years later (Brown et al 1981).

While not included in his classification, MacNaughton-Jones alluded in various parts of his book to psychological factors in tinnitus, even indicating that the only times that he himself suffered from the symptom had been when he was under considerable stress.

He also advocates massage (Fig. 1.6a) and tapotement (Fig. 1.6b) for the treatment of tinnitus, commenting 'I do not pretend to explain how it acts, but it has in some cases decidely beneficial effect'. Furthermore, presumably related to his well-to-do clientéle, he advocates spa treatment for many of his patients, the choice of spa being dependent on the aetiology of the tinnitus.

At one point he was even prepared to stick his neck out with a chapter entitled 'Prognosis' giving two lists of causes of tinnitus, those with a poor prognosis and those with a good prognosis. It is difficult to generalize about the two groups and there is even some overlap between the two. However, on the whole those with a good prognosis tended to be the obstructive peripheral conditions and acute disorders, whereas those with a poor prognosis were the chronic and systemic conditions. Chronic Ménière's disease was included among those with a poor prognosis, and ototoxic effects with a good prognosis. This latter is probably due to the fact that at the time the main antibacterial drugs, arsenicals and aminoglycoside antibiotics, had not been discovered and the well-known ototoxics which he listed, salicin and quinine, are still considered generally to have reversible effects. Even before MacNaughton-Jones' time, Maillard (1880) had demonstrated such reversibility in their effects on the auditory threshold (Stephens 1982).

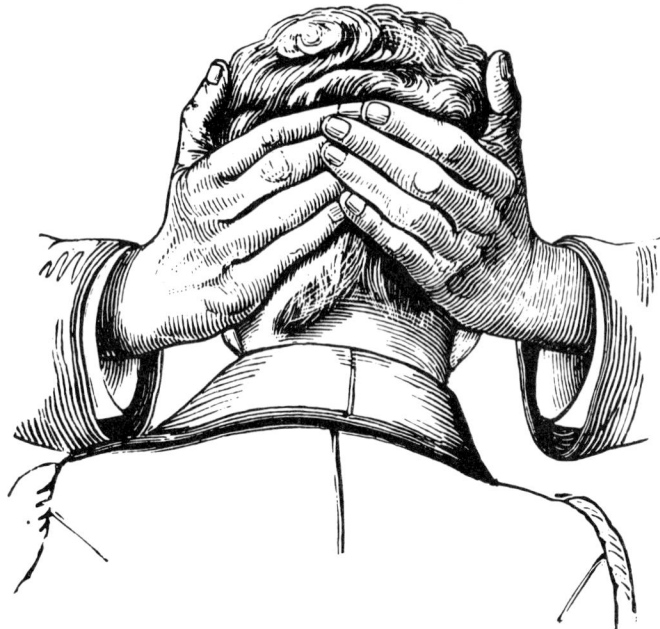

Fig. 1.6a Massage for tinnitus. (Reproduced with permission from MacNaughton Jones 1891.)

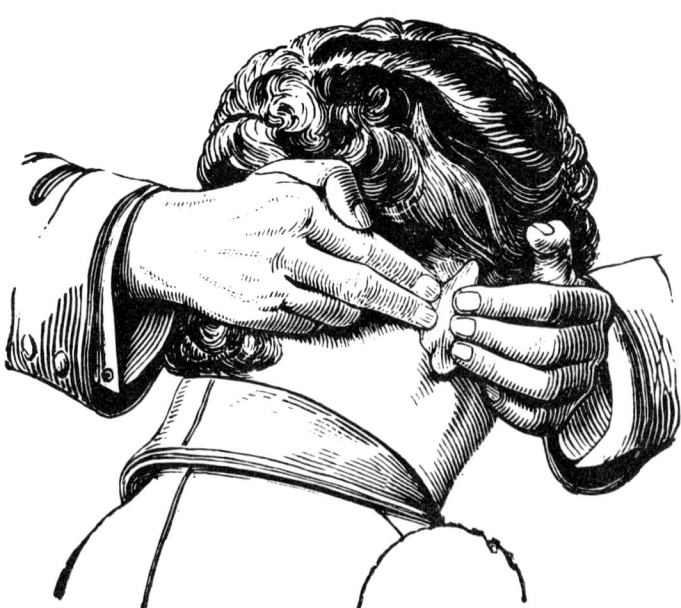

Fig. 1.6b Tapotement for tinnitus. (Reproduced with permission from MacNaughton Jones 1891.)

MacNaughton-Jones made no reference to the masking of tinnitus and the work of Itard (1821) seems to have been ignored or unknown. A couple of years later the American Harold Wilson (1893) described a technique recalling that of Wepfer (1727) in which he attempted to suppress the tinnitus by exposing the ears to a clicking noise produced electrically in a telephone. The results of this approach were not particularly impressive even in his initial presentation, and the technique does not appear to have been widely adopted. Masking was alluded to only in passing in Spalding's publication (1903), mainly concerned with the musical description of tinnitus, and the first electrical tinnitus-masking device was developed by Jones & Knudsen in 1928, their harmonic generator (Fig. 1.7). It is, however, interesting to note, for example, that although the first edition of Porter's textbook published in 1912 made no reference to the masking of tinnitus, the second edition published in 1916 (with the collaboration of McBride) included the statement 'it has also been suggested to make the patient sleep in a noisy room, or to place a loud ticking clock near his bed', so rediscovering, or at least reiterating, Itard's suggestions.

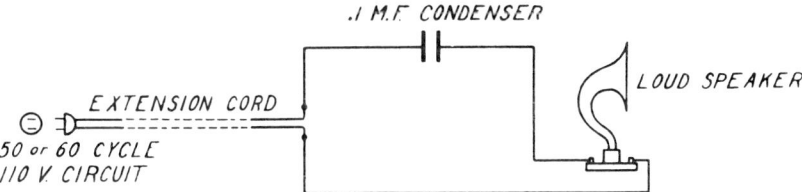

Fig. 1.7 Diagram of Jones and Knudsen's (1928) harmonic generator for tinnitus masking.

20TH CENTURY

A variety of other surgical and pharmacological treatments for tinnitus were described in the late 19th and early 20th century and some have been discussed elsewhere (Stephens 1986). None, however, have stood the test of time. From then through to the present day there was little development until the upsurge of interest in tinnitus in the past decade. The results of the latter are described elsewhere in this volume.

There are, however, two exceptions to this hiatus, the demonstration by Saltzman & Ersner (1947) of the effectiveness of hearing aids in suppressing tinnitus, and the examination of the psychological factors associated with tinnitus by Fowler (1948).

CONCLUSION

Many famous and infamous people from Martin Luther to Adolf Hitler (Irving 1983) and from Jean-Jacques Rousseau to Goya and Smetana have suffered from tinnitus and this has arguably had a significant influence on their work and behaviour. To consider all such cases and their possible influences on the development of literature, art, music, religion or even of the history of mankind itself, would require a book in itself. It is, however, perhaps salutory to conclude by recalling the case of the great pioneer of the study of the pathology of ear disease, Joseph Toynbee (1815-1866). On July 7 1866, believing that tinnitus might be relieved by inhalation of the vapours of chloroform and prussic acid, with subsequent Valsalva inflation, he subjected himself to the test, with fatal results (Stevenson & Guthrie 1949). He may thus be honoured as the first known martyr of tinnitus research.

Acknowledgements

I am grateful to Dick Hallam, Simon Jakes and Tony Wright for their invaluable comments during the preparation of this manuscript.

REFERENCES

Adams F 1844 The seven books of Paulus Aegineta. Sydenham Society, London
Avicenna 1964 Libera canonis (1964 edn.). Georg Olms, Hildesheim
Asherson N 1979 Traité de l'organ de l'ouie. Journal of Laryngology and Otology, Supplement 2
Bacon F 1627 Sylva Sylvarum. Rawley, London
Bartel M 1893 Die medizin der Naturvölker. Leipzig
Bolland J J 1694 Disputatio inauguralis medica de tinnitu aurium. Krebs, Jena
Brenner R 1868 Untersuchungen und Beobachtungen auf dem Gebiete der Elektrotherapie. Giesecke und Devrient, Leipzig
Brown R D, Penny J E, Henley C M et al 1981 Ototoxic drugs and noise. In: Evered D, Lawrenson G (eds) Tinnitus. Ciba Foundation Symposium 85. Pitman, London, pp 150–165
Campbell Thompson R 1931 Assyrian prescriptions for diseases of the ears. Journal of the Royal Asiatic Society, pp 1–25
Cartheuser J F 1770 Dissertationem de susurratione et tinnitus aurium. Frankfurt
Du Verney J G 1683 Traité de l'organ de l'ouie. Michallet, Paris
Du Verney J G 1737 A treatise of the organ of hearing. Baker, London
Fallopio G 1563 De morbo Gallico. Gryphium, Padua

Feldmann H 1984 Suppression of tinnitus by electrical stimulation: a contribution to the history of medicine. Journal of Laryngology and Otology Supplement 9: 123–124
Forster E S 1927 Problemata. In: Ross W D (ed) The works of Aristotle. Clarendon, Oxford
Fowler E P 1948 The emotional factor in tinnitus aurium. Laryngoscope 58: 145–154.
Garrison F H 1929 An introduction to the history of medicine, 4th edn. Saunders, Philadelphia
Getz F M 1981 An edition of the Middle English Gilbertus Anglicus found in Wellcome MS 537. Unpublished PhD Thesis, University of Toronto
Grapengeisser C J C 1801 Versuche den Galvanismus zur Heilung einiger Krankheiten. Myliussischen, Berlin
Guerrier Y, Mounier-Kuhn P 1980 Histoire des maladies de l'oreille, du nez et de la gorge. Dacosta, Paris
Guirand F 1959 Assyro–Babylonian mythology. In: New Larousse Encyclopaedia of Mythology. Hamlyn, London
Hartmann M 1669 Dissertationem inauguralem medicam de tinnitu aurium. Krebs, Jena
Irving D 1983 Adolf Hitler medical diaries. Sidgwick and Jackson, London
Itard J M G 1821 Traité des maladies de l'oreille et de l'audition. Mequignon–Marvis, Paris
Jones I H, Knudsen V O 1928 Certain aspects of tinnitus, particularly treatment. Laryngoscope 38: 597–611
Kamal H 1968 Dictionary of Pharaonic medicine. National Publication House, Cairo
King-Hele D 1981 The letters of Erasmus Darwin. Cambridge University Press, Cambridge
Kuhn C G 1965 Claudii Galeni opera omnia. Georg Olms, Hildesheim
Lane H 1976 The wild boy of Aveyron. Harvard University Press, Cambridge, Mass.
Leca A-P 1971 La médicine Egyptienne. Dacosta, Paris

Leschevin 1776 Memoire sur la théorie des maladies de l'oreille. Mémoires de l'Academié Royale de Chirurgie 4: 677
Littré E 1840 Oeuvres complètes d'Hippocrate. Baillière, Paris
MacNaughton Jones H 1891 Subjective noises in the head and ears: their etiology, diagnosis and treatment. Baillière, Tindall and Cox, London
Maillard C 1880 L'audiomètre et ses applications. Thèse, Université de Nacy Première serie No 111
Müller J 1834-40 Handbuch der Physiologie des Menschen. Holscher, Coblenz
Ogden M S 1971 The Cyrurgie of Guy de Chauliac. Oxford University Press, London
Opsomer-Halleux C 1981 Le nez, la gorge et les oreilles dan les manuscrits médicaux de l'antiquité et du moyen áge (réceptaires et antidotaires). Acta Oto-Rhino-Laryngologica Belgica 35, Supplement 4: 1583–1599
Politzer A 1907 Geschichte der Ohrenheilkunde. Vol. 1. Enke Verlag, Stuttgart
Porter W G 1912 Diseases of the throat, nose, and ear for practitioners and students. Wright, Bristol
Porter W G, McBride P 1916 Diseases of the throat, nose, and ear for practitioners and students, 2nd edn. Wright, Bristol
Reymond E A E 1976 A medical book from Crocodilopolis. Hollinek, Vienna
Saltzman M, Ersner M S 1947 A hearing aid for the relief of tinnitus aurium. Laryngoscope 57: 358-366
Spalding J A 1903 Tinnitus, with a plea for its more accurate musical notation. Annals of Otology 32: 272
Spencer W G 1938 Celsus 'De medicina'. Heinemann, London
Stephens S D G 1981 L'audiométrie—un aperçu historique. Acta Oto-Rhino-Laryngologica Belgica 35: Supplement 4: 1399–1425
Stephens S D G 1982 Some historical aspects of ototoxicity. British Journal of Audiology 16: 76-80
Stephens S D G 1984 The treatment of tinnitus—a historical perspective. Journal of Laryngology and Otology 98: 963–972
Stephens S D G 1986 The management of tinnitus. Paper to the International Workshop Symposium on Neuro-otology, Asiago, Italy, January 1984. Audiologia Italiana (in press)
Stephens S D G, Goodwin J C 1984 Non-electric aids to hearing: a short history. Audiology 23: 215–240
Stevenson R S, Guthrie D 1949 A history of oto-laryngology. Livingstone, Edinburgh
Volta A 1800 On the electricity excited by mere contact of the conducting substances of different kinds. Philosophical Transactions of the Royal Society 90: 403–431
Wepfer J J 1727 Observationes medico-practicae de affectibus capitis internis et externis. Ziegler, Schaffhausen
Wibel G D 1768 Casum aegroti auditu difficili. Heitzii, Strasbourg
Wilde W 1853 Practical observations on aural surgery and the nature and treatment of diseases of the ear. Churchill, London
Wilson H 1893 Vibratory massage of the middle ear by means of the telephone. New York Medical Journal 57:221–222
Wright A 1985 Structural changes in the human cochlea during treament. Unpublished MD Thesis, University of Oxford

Theory of tinnitus generation

J. P. Wilson

This chapter will consider the way in which acoustic signals are received and analysed by the ear and then processed by the brain to give rise to the sensation of hearing. It is when something goes wrong in this chain of events that we may perceive sound when no appropriate external source is present. There are many levels at which malfunction could occur and therefore many different possible origins of tinnitus. Although the periphery is much better understood than the more central processes, our conception of how the inner ear works has changed dramatically within the last few years. This has not as yet given us much insight into the mechanisms of tinnitus generation apart from that related to otoacoustic emissions; animal models, however, are giving promising clues to other sources of tinnitus. Various malfunctions possibly responsible for tinnitus will be discussed below, against the background of the normal auditory function of each stage of the system.

SOUND RECEPTION AND TRANSMISSION

The external ear

The external ear, or pinna, acts as a funnel or horn which partly matches the low acoustic impedance* of air to the much higher impedance of the fluid-filled cochlea. It tends to reinforce mid- to high-frequency sounds arriving at about 45° from the front in the horizontal plane. More importantly, its convoluted form reflects and diffracts the higher frequency components of sound, causing interference between the various soundpaths and subtle changes in the spectrum of sound frequencies passing into the ear canal. This spectral change is different for different directions of sound source and acts as a clue to direction. This spectral labelling is the chief reason why normal sounds appear to be out in space whereas headphone sounds, or internally generated signals such as tinnitus, appear to be within the ears or head. Although these spectral clues are restricted to the higher frequencies, low-frequency components of the same complex sound appear to be located at the same place. The second ear, at a different position in space, and pointing in a different direction, will have a different spectral tag which the brain uses to reinforce this information.

---

* There are different definitions of impedance for different systems, but it can be thought of as the force or pressure required to produce a certain velocity of movement.

Furthermore, the differences between the two ears in sound intensity and time of arrival provide the familiar binaural or 'stereo' clues to direction and help greatly in separating wanted signals from background noises (the 'cocktail-party effect').

The ear canal

The outer ear, or ear canal, both provides mechanical protection for the delicate middle and inner ear mechanisms and acts as an open-pipe resonator. This further improves the acoustic impedance matching between the air and the cochlea, increasing the sensitivity at the resonance frequency of 3–4 kHz, and thereby providing the lowest free-field threshold of about 20 μPa (0 dB SPL*). This is an important region for speech intelligibility but the high sensitivity also increases the risk of noise damage and may be responsible for the frequent finding of a notch at 4 kHz. This pathology is a very frequent presumed cause of tinnitus, which could have been avoided by the use of hearing protection. Unfortunately, many of the powerful loudspeakers used in sound amplification tend to have resonance peaks in the same frequency region.

The ear canal is a potential repository for wax and foreign matter. This has several possible implications for tinnitus such as friction noises, and blockage of the ear canal which could render internal noises more audible because the masking effects of external sounds are reduced. The occlusion effect of Békésy (1960) may increase the loudness of bone-conducted sounds with a blockage of the ear canal, whereas the inertia effect (Tonndorf 1966) may be reduced by stiffening of the middle ear. Sources of tinnitus influenced by these factors can be either objective, such as blood flow, muscular activity, Eustachian tube clicks, spontaneous otoacoustic emissions (SOAEs), or intrinsic to the nervous system. The altered acoustic impedance of the middle ear may also initiate or alter the generation of SOAEs (see below).

The middle ear

The middle ear performs two important functions in the acoustic process. Firstly, it acts as an impedance transformer between the air and the fluids of the cochlea and secondly, it is under muscular control which can afford some protection for the cochlea from certain loud sounds.

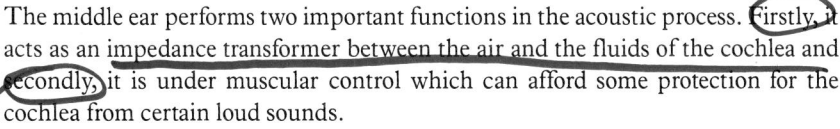

The impedance transformation (supplemented as mentioned above, at higher frequencies by the pinna and ear canal) is achieved in two ways. Firstly, by the mechanical lever action of the ossicles which is about 1.3:1 in man and secondly, and much more substantially, by the pressure amplification produced by the force acting on the large area of the tympanic membrane being concentrated on the small piston area of the stapes (a ratio of about 17:1 in man (Békésy 1960, for other contributory factors see Tonndorf & Khanna 1970)). Unfortunately, the middle ear cannot be massless (weightless), even though the ossicles have a remarkable geometry to minimise the influence of mass without losing rigidity, nor can it be suspended without constraint, which introduces stiffness. The effective (moving) mass and

* SPL = sound pressure level.

effective stiffness act together to produce a mechanical resonance* at about 1.2 kHz in man. At resonance the effects of mass and stiffness cancel out and allow the most efficient flow of energy through the middle ear. At lower frequencies the effects of stiffness, and at higher frequencies the effects of mass, predominate and progressively reduce the efficiency of transmission of acoustic energy. Any energy that is not transmitted is partly absorbed by the middle ear, but mostly reflected back into the ear canal, or (for sound that originates within the inner ear: see p. 00 below), back into the cochlea.

The role of the middle ear muscles in protection from loud sounds, and in compressing the dynamic range, is still not well understood. It is clear that a simple stiffening influence will raise the resonance frequency and reduce the response to all frequencies below resonance. Békésy (1960) has suggested that at very high sound levels the mode of transmission may be altered. The tensing of the stapedius muscle is generally considered to produce the acoustic reflex for certain sounds above about 70-90 dB SPL in normal ears. Not only is the maximum degree of protection restricted and confined to lower frequencies, but it will not be rapid enough to attenuate impulsive sounds and it will adapt (i.e. become progressively less effective) to sustained sounds. Perhaps the predominant function is protection from self-vocalised sounds which can be anticipated by the nervous system.

The middle ear can be implicated in tinnitus in several ways. It is common in otosclerosis, and is a cardinal symptom in glomus jugulare tumours. Blood flow in overlying or nearby vessels can produce heart-beat noises or pulsed rushing noises. The author has recorded pulsed broad-band noises, that were audible to the subject, which are presumed to be due to blood flow. Whistles have also been reported (see Glanville et al 1971) but it is now thought that these may be SOAEs (Wilson & Sutton 1983, see below). The middle-ear muscles also spontaneously produce a high level of low-frequency noise, predominantly in the 10 Hz region, which can be detected by a microphone, and may be very audible to some subjects as tensor tympani syndrome (Klochoff 1981). Certain complaints of 'hum' may originate in this way (Walford 1983). Voluntary contraction of the middle ear muscles can greatly enhance this effect and produce a rumbling sound.

The middle ear is also implicated in the SOAE generation process (see below) by virtue of the impedance it presents to the cochlea. It may, under normal conditions, reflect sufficient acoustic energy back into the cochlea to maintain SOAEs, or it may do so only under abnormal conditions which stiffen the system, e.g., external or middle ear pressure, or otosclerosis. A fairly common report is that movement of the jaw either initiates or modifies tinnitus. Presumably this either acts directly, mechanically on the middle ear, or initiates corollary contraction of the middle-ear muscles. The author has seen one case in which tinnitus could be initiated by jaw movement, and several in which tinnitus could be modified, in which the observations were confirmed by corresponding signals from a sealed-in microphone.

---

* A system moves with maximum velocity at its resonance frequency, with progressively less motion for lower or higher frequencies. Such a system is therefore 'tuned' to its resonance frequency, and can be considered as a filter maximally sensitive to its resonance frequency and less sensitive to others.

We have, however, so far failed to find any converse case in which persistent tinnitus could be reliably stopped by adjustment of the external ear pressure.

The Eustachian tube allows the pressure inside the middle ear to be maintained at atmospheric pressure. There are four ways in which its malfunction can influence tinnitus. 1. Chronic blockage will allow the air within the cavity to be absorbed, building up a negative pressure. This will displace the eardrum and stapes inwards, stiffening it and giving rise to the problems discussed above. 2. A build-up of middle-ear fluid will also stiffen up the middle ear and lead to a similar result. 3. The opening and closing of the Eustachian tube is a common source of clicking sounds within the ear. 4. A patulous Eustachian tube will allow some sound cancellation at lower frequencies, and allow internal sounds to enter the middle-ear cavity (O'Connor & Shea 1981).

The inner ear

Our understanding of how the cochlea functions has increased greatly in recent years although there are still areas of considerable uncertainty and controversy. In a sense the classical viewpoint of hydro-mechanical frequency analysis producing an ordered stimulation of the end organ of hair cells is still correct, but the way in which this is achieved is much more ingenious than previously thought. In particular it appears that the end organ itself plays an active role in the mechanical processes. Furthermore, it is now clear from animal experiments that there are several mechanisms by which frequency analysis takes place. Some of these may be specific to certain classes of animals but it cannot yet be ruled out that several mechanisms may be involved, to some degree, in human hearing.

Passive basilar membrane mechanics

The classical Helmholtz model was that the basilar membrane (BM) acted like a series of strings stretched across its width, having graded lengths and tensions. Each string acted as an independent resonator vibrating maximally and stimulating its receptor when the incoming sound was tuned to it. Békésy (1953) showed a somewhat different type of motion, which he described as a travelling wave (Fig. 2.1).

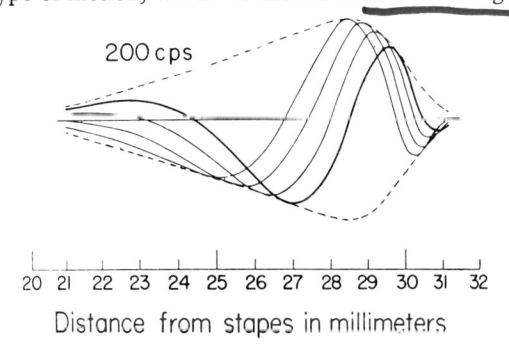

Fig. 2.1 A travelling wave of basilar membrane (BM) displacement at four successive times along a human cochlear partition in response to a 200 Hz tone. The travelling wave remains within the envelope indicated by the dashed lines and would be transposed towards the left (base) or right (apex) for higher and lower frequencies respectively. (From Békésy 1953).

Unfortunately the measured sharpness of tuning of this was found to be inadequate to explain either psychophysical tuning or the more recently reported single cochlear nerve fibre tuning (Kiang et al 1965, Evans 1975). Békésy attempted to overcome this discrepancy by invoking lateral inhibition to sharpen up the response. Although there were problems with this type of solution, it led to a whole series of attempts to identify what became known as the 'second' filter (Evans & Wilson 1973). In mammals this search has partly ended with the discovery of active mechanical processes, discussed below. The passive travelling wave has been measured in a large number of species. Békésy (1960) observed it in the apical, or low-frequency, half of the cochlea in the chicken, the mouse, the rat, the cow, the elephant and more extensively in the guinea pig and man. Using the Mössbauer technique, Johnstone et al (1970) were able to show that tuning of the BM is somewhat sharper at the basal end in the guinea pig. Rhode (1971, 1978) was able to show even sharper tuning at the 7 kHz position in the squirrel monkey. Although not recognised as such at the time, these were probably the first results to show some influence of active mechanisms. Wilson & Johnstone (1975) extended the range of positions on the guinea pig BM at SPLs down to 40 dB. Evans & Wilson (1975) were able to measure concurrently from ostensibly the same place on cat BM, sharp single cochlear nerve fibre responses and the typical, much poorer, passive BM tuning—apparently proof of the need for a second filter (but see discussion of active mechanical processes below). Passive BM mechanics were reported more extensively in the cat by Wilson & Evans (1983a), in the greater horseshoe bat (Wilson & Burns 1983) which is notable for its extremely sharp neural tuning (Suga et al 1976), and in the caiman alligator (Wilson et al 1985). All these animals have qualitatively very similar BM responses. Not all animals follow this pattern however. The alligator lizard has an oval BM which appears to be untuned relative to its middle ear (Weiss et al 1978). Even more different, anurans (frogs and toads) have hair cells that are rigidly supported within their hearing organs (basilar papilla, amphibian papilla, sacculus) with no analogue of the BM (Wever 1978).

Over the years a large number of attempts have been made to model the behaviour of the BM with varying degrees of success. We shall not review these but simply state that they have included hydromechanical, electrical, computer and analytical models, in one, two or three dimensions (see de Boer 1980) which together have provided a good understanding of the system. For present purposes it is sufficiently accurate to assume that they represent a series of coupled resonators, where the mass is provided by the cochlear partition, and does not vary much with longitudinal position, and the stiffness is provided chiefly by the BM itself, which is wider and thinner at the apical end. The coupling is provided mostly by the fluid rather than the longitudinal stiffness of the BM. The system is heavily damped by the BM and the fluid and so is incapable of possessing sharp tuning.

The end result of a system in which the resonance frequency of neighbouring elements becomes progressively lower, the further we move along the system, is a travelling wave (Fig. 2.1). For a single pure tone simulation, a maximal response is obtained near the point of resonance. This will be near the base for high frequencies and towards the apex for low frequencies. The amplitude of upward and downward motion of the BM will decrease gradually towards the base and more rapidly towards the apex giving an asymmetrical response. Within this overall envelope of vibration, individual waves will appear at the base and move continuously, but progressively more slowly, towards the apex. As each wave disappears apically a new one will be starting basally. The total number of waves visible within the envelope will depend upon the model, or upon the species, and on the frequency; values between 0.5 and 3.5 waves have been observed. The pattern is likely to be very different when active mechanisms are involved (see below). It should be noted that the simultaneous presence of upward and downward displacement implies a high degree of cancellation in the net displacement of the BM. The residue is provided by the piston displacement of the stapes. This effect explains how, with incompressible fluid, the maximum BM amplitude can be typically thirty times greater than the stapes displacement (and much more than this with active processes). This aspect is also relevant to the reverse process in which sound generated within the inner ear (e.g. SOAEs) can find its way into the ear canal. It will be the total net volume displacement within scala vestibuli and scala media that will react back on the stapes, whereas it will be the local amplitude or velocity of motion which stimulates the individual hair cells.

Active mechanical processes

In an active system, amplification of the input energy takes place, and the properties of the system can be modified greatly by feeding back part of the output into the input. If the feedback is negative as in many electronic amplifiers the performance can be improved in many ways, at the cost of reduced overall gain. For a given level of output the non-linear distortion can be reduced by the same factor as the feedback, and the band-width increased. For a second-order (e.g. mass and stiffness controlled) system, increased band-width is equivalent to the effects of increased damping in the system. Entirely the opposite effects can be produced by positive feedback, which at first sight might be thought to be undesirable. It can, however, be used to overcome the effects of damping and increase the gain and sharpness of tuning of a system. Unfortunately, however, as positive feedback is increased, instability, in the form of continuous oscillation, results (see below).

Gold (1948) first postulated that the cochlea employs positive mechanical feedback to overcome the inherent damping and sharpen up its tuning. This view was not taken seriously at the time, partly because his assumptions were based, unrealistically, on a simple second-order resonator, but more particularly because it was felt that the inherent problems of instability would be insuperable for the system. Until very recently direct BM measurements appeared to support this view. The first experimental evidence suggesting active mechanical processes, however, was that of otoacoustic emissions (OAEs) (Kemp 1978) discussed below. The earlier mechanical measurements of Rhode (1971, 1978) on the squirrel monkey BM did, however, point in this direction. The decisive evidence came from Khanna & Leonard (1982) and Sellick et al (1982), who showed in the cat (Fig. 2.2) and the guinea pig respectively, BM responses which approached neural responses in terms of sharpness of tuning. The two groups interpret their data differently. Khanna (1983) suggests that the sharp

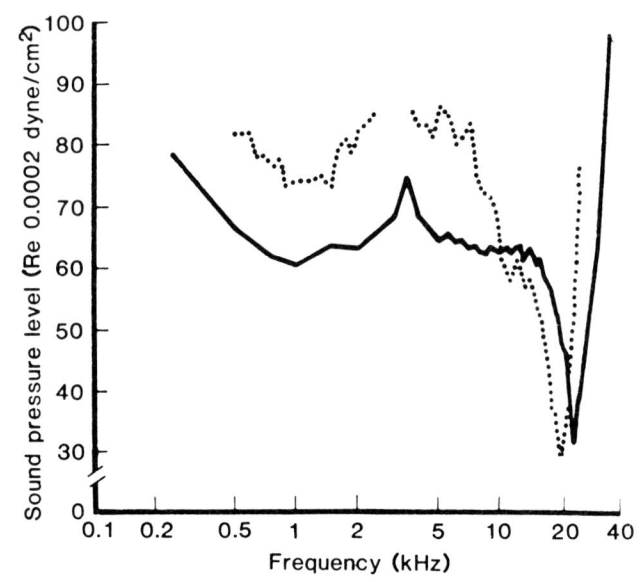

Fig. 2.2 BM tuning curve (solid line, representing SPL as a function of frequency, producing BM vibration amplitude of 0.3 nm) compared with a neural tuning curve (dotted line, representing SPL producing an increase in firing rate by 10 spikes/s) from the basal region of cat cochlea (from Khanna & Leonard 1982). This sharp BM tuning implies active mechanical processes (see text) and that the travelling wave of Fig. 2.1 would be much sharper in an intact cochlea.

mechanical resonator lies in the hair cell stereocilia bundles and can be seen reflected in the BM response when all hair cells are fully functional. He does not specifically invoke active mechanisms, and does not attribute different functions and properties to the inner and outer hair cells (ihc, ohc). Johnstone (1983), however, presents evidence and suggests that neural and BM tuning should be identical and implies that the inner hair cells are passive, and untuned, receptors of BM motion. It is also implied that the ohcs provide the active mechanism to sharpen up the BM response.

Gross electrical recordings from the cochlea

Although recording from electrodes within the scalae and on the surface of the cochlea have given considerable insight into its function (see Dallos 1975), some of the results have also tended to be misleading.

The d.c. electrical potentials within various compartments depend upon ionic composition and active ion-transport mechanisms. If the perilymph (high Na^+, low K^+) is taken as reference (0 mV), the endolymph (low Na^+, high K^+) has a potential of +80 mV (due to the ion pumping properties of the stria vascularis, which acts as an electrical battery), and the hair cells have an internal potential of about -40 mV. According to the Davis (1965) model, mechanical bending of the stereocilia alters the electrical resistance of the upper end of the hair cell and modulates the current flow through it, which in turn leads to chemical transmitter release at its lower end, which initiates nerve impulses.

Stimulation of the ear with sound leads to three gross electrical components, the cochlear microphonic (CM), the summating potential (SP), and the action potential (AP). The CM appears as an electrical version of the signal waveform, which is frequency-filtered according to the position of the electrodes, and limited in amplitude according to frequency and SPL. The best attempts to obtain localised pick-up using differential electrodes, however, fail to show any sharper tuning than the classical passive mechanical BM response. If the intact BM is vibrating in a sharply-tuned manner, it is difficult to imagine how a truly local CM could fail to be equally sharply tuned. It would seem either that even the best attempts at obtaining a localised response in fact average over a large number of hair cells tuned to different frequencies, which thereby mimics the poor tuning of the passive BM or, less likely, that *all* such attempts have damaged the cochlea.

The SP appears to be a non-linear d.c. component arising from the rectifier-action of the hair cell transduction process and at the local level may have an important role in transmitter release, perhaps particularly at higher frequencies where the hair cell may be less able to follow the stimulus waveform.

The AP, on the other hand, appears to be a post-synaptic potential resulting from synchronised firing of a number of nerve fibres. Unlike the CM and SP, it appears to have a definite threshold and this can be used as a monitor of the physiological condition of the cochlea. Although much easier to obtain, none of these potentials is as informative about cochlear function as the individual unit responses. The latter can be recorded either extra-or intra-cellularly, or from cochlear nerve fibres.

Although abnormalities in the electrical condition of the cochlea would seem to be a likely cause for tinnitus, there is so far little evidence for this occurring naturally. Electrical stimulation, however, can influence tinnitus (Cazals et al 1978, see also Ch. 6). Pulses, as well as d.c. polarisation, appear to be effective. Negative pulses at the round window, or scala tympani, frequently give auditory sensation (the basis of cochlear implants) whereas positive pulses appear to suppress tinnitus in many patients. The implications of this would appear to be that spontaeous activity in cochlear nerve fibres might be reduced by this procedure, contrary to the implications of some of the animal models (see below).

Hair cell responses

Recordings from individual inner hair cells were first made by Russel & Sellick (1978) and these were found to be as sharply tuned as single cochlear nerve fibres (see below). Both a.c. and d.c. components were recorded. The properties of the d.c. component would appear to be appropriate for it to be the generator of the SP (see above). For the cells with higher CFs, from which Russell and Sellick recorded, the a.c. component appears to be attenuated both within the hair cell, because of the cell membrane capacitance, and also by the recording electrode, because of its high internal resistance and the capacitive shunting due to the surrounding fluids. The position with regard to outer hair cell responses is less clear. There are a number of reasons for expecting them to be equally sharply tuned, and recent measurements have confirmed this (Dallos 1985). Although traditionally the ohcs have been considered to be more sensitive, it is now thought that ihcs and ohcs perform different functions. Crawford & Fettiplace (1981) demonstrated that in the turtle, unlike mammals, the hair-cell tuning is electrical.

Anatomy and innervation of the cochlea

The structure of the organ of Corti is complex (Fig. 2.3). It is thought that the stereocilia of the outer hair cells are embedded in the tectorial membrane, but in some species at least, the inner hair cell stereocilia are free-standing (Lim 1980). The classical model is that as the BM is displaced, it bends the stereocilia against the tectorial membrane. Recent findings of active mechanical processes imply that the matter is considerably more complicated. One such possibility is that the ohc stereocilia might be motile, reacting both on the BM via the cell bodies, and on the ihc via the tectorial membrane. Another possibility, suggested by the findings of Brownell et al (1985), discussed below, is that the ohc may show length vibrations, which again may react on the BM and on the stereocilia/tectorial membrane interface.

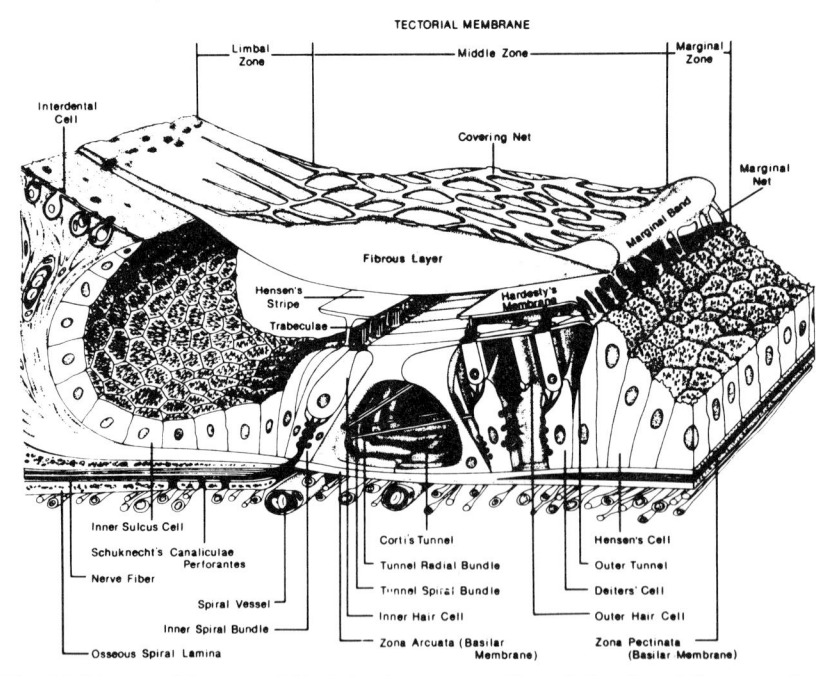

Fig. 2.3 Diagram of the organ of Corti showing one row of inner hair cells and three rows of outer hair cells in relation to the tectorial membrane (from Lim 1980).

The innervation pattern of the inner and outer hair cells is quite different (Spoendlin 1967). 90–95% of the afferent fibres arise from the inner cells with 20–30 unbranched fibres from each cell. The fibres from the outer hair cells, however, pick up from several cells over a range of about 0.2 mm, then descend in an apical direction for about 0.5–0.7 mm between the supporting pillar cells until they reach the BM. They then turn and cross the tunnel of Corti in a radial direction and pass into the spiral lamina via openings of the habenula perforata. Within the spiral lamina of the modiolus lies the spiral array of afferent cell bodies—the spiral ganglion.

The efferent innervation also goes to both inner and outer hair cells, via the inner spiral bundle, onto the ihc afferent dendrites, and high across the tunnel of Corti with terminal branching onto several ochs.

Unit responses from the cochlea

The properties of single cochlear nerve fibres have been extensively described by Kiang et al (1965) in the cat and these results have since been confirmed and greatly extended by many groups in a number of species. Only a brief summary can be given here (for review see Evans 1975). In mammals most or all fibres are spontaneously active (0–80 spikes/s) in the absence of sound. When stimulated with lower frequencies the random (Poisson) activity tends to become phase-locked to the stimulus and for all frequencies the mean rate of discharge increases up to a saturation level. A refractory or recovery period of about 1 ms limits the maximum rate of impulses to several hundred per second, although owing to adaptation, the saturation rate decreases with time. Most fibres show a restricted dynamic range of 20–50 dB above threshold and most unit thresholds lie close to the behavioural audiogram. Individual fibres are tuned to different frequencies (CFs) over the range from about 50 Hz to near the upper limit of hearing of the animal (Fig. 2.4). The tuning curve of an individual fibre represents the boundary between spontaneous and driven activity and rises (i.e. becomes less sensitive) towards lower and higher frequencies. For lower CFs, on a log frequency scale, the curves are symmetrical with slopes of about 30 dB/octave whereas above 2 kHz they are asymmetrical with steeper

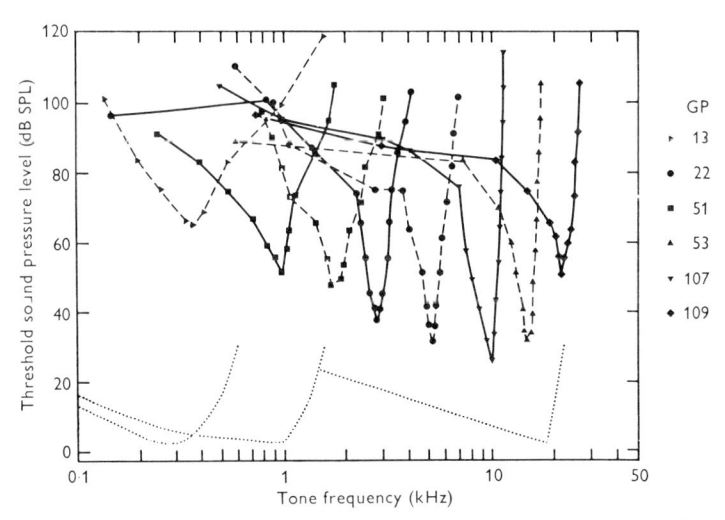

Fig. 2.4 Frequency threshold (tuning) curves from eight cochlear nerve fibres in the guinea pig compared with BM tuning (dotted lines, arbitrary ordinate). SPLs and frequencies within (i.e. above) the tuning curves produce increased firing rates in that fibre. The envelope of the lowest thresholds (at CF) of all fibres represents approximately the audiogram of that animal (from Evans 1972).

high-frequency slopes (100-1000 dB/octave) and only a limited range of steep (100–200 dB/octave) low frequency cut-off. Below this there is a tail segment of lower slope with low sensitivity to low-frequency stimulation (Fig. 2.4). The filter shape represented by the tuning curve shows linear behaviour to some stimuli and non-linear behaviour to others. Techniques for deriving the shape of the filter characteristics at higher sound levels show that it changes only slightly with level, eventually becoming broader with a slight shift in CF. The neural response behaves non-linearly, however, in the presence of a second tone which can suppress the response to the first (two-tone suppression, 2TS) and in responding to intermodulation products (e.g. a fibre tuned to the frequency $2f_1-f_2$, will respond as if energy is present at the frequency even though the stimulus contains only the frequencies f_1 and f_2 and the fibre will not respond to either f_1 or f_2 alone).

Similar responses have been obtained from spiral ganglion cells (Robertson & Manley 1974). This has the advantage of knowing either approximately, or in the case of horseradish peroxidase neurone tracing (Liberman 1982) exactly, at which point along the cochlear partition responses arise and thereby reveals the cochlear frequency map. It also has the advantage of easier attainment of stable recordings than with fibres, but it does involve opening the cochlea and thereby increasing the chance of damage. The implications of abnormalities in hair cells and in neural responses will be discussed below.

Neural pathways

The central pathways are complex (Fig 2.5) and not well understood, with many possibilities for interaction between the left and right pathways and between higher and lower levels (see Aitkin & Webster 1984). The main pathway is contralateral from the antero-ventral cochlear nucleus (AVCN), via the trapezoid body to the contralateral superior olivary complex (SOC) and upwards, and also, from the posterioventral cochlear nucleus (PVCN) and dorsal cochlear nucleus (DCN) to the contralateral lateral lemniscus and nucleus of lateral lemniscus, inferior colliculus, medial geniculate body, and cortex. The ipsilateral pathway is via AVCN, SOC, inferior colliculus, medial geniculate body, and cortex.

The way in which the central nervous system represents stimuli is still controversial. The 'feature-detector' viewpoint would be that activity in a single cell might represent a quite complex and specific percept. The alternative view is that perception arises by virtue of the pattern of activity over many cells. Although a strict interpretation of the former view now appears unlikely, the responses do become more complex and mean firing rates become lower as signals ascend in the system, owing to the opposing effects of excitation and inhibition between cells. In addition to the main afferent pathways there are the main descending pathways and many minor ones. The main peripheral efferent pathway to the cochlea is represented by the crossed olivo-cochlear bundle.

On the two models it would appear that a malfunction might have rather different consequences for tinnitus. Activity of a feature detector, for example, would be expected to lead to perception of that feature, however it was stimulated. At higher

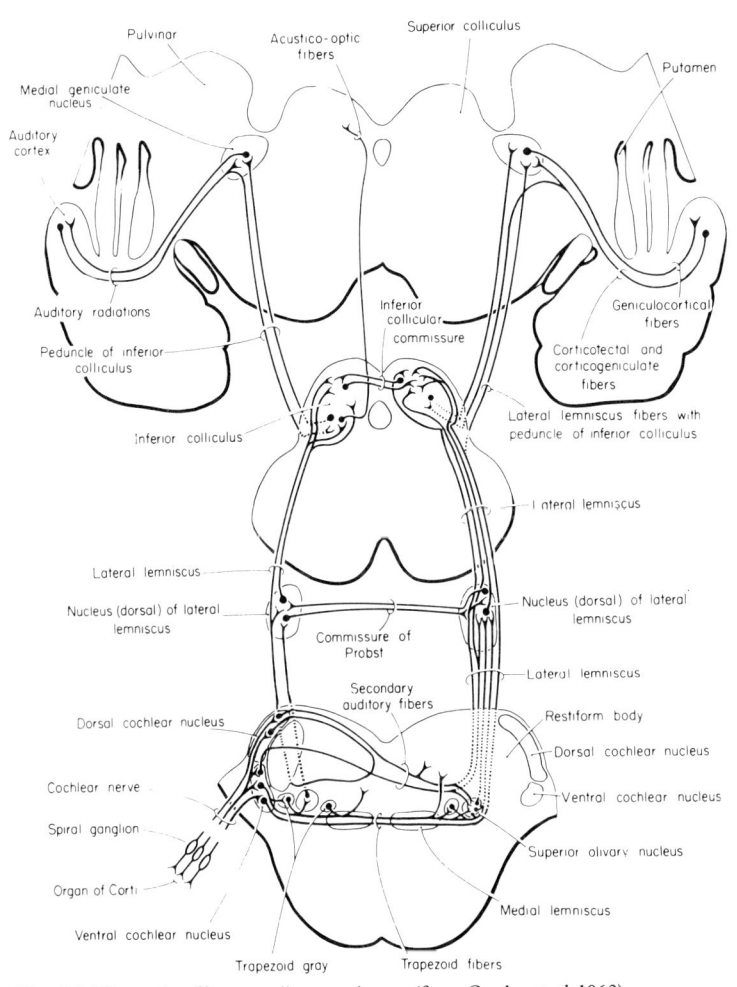

Fig. 2.5 The main afferent auditory pathways (from Crosby et al 1962)

levels, few feature detectors would be expected to be devoted to relatively simple stimuli such as tinnitus. Thus on this model, the initial neural activity giving rise to tinnitus would be expected to be limited to locations which were quite peripheral. This restriction might be less obvious where the overall pattern of activity is involved. Even with this model, however, it is intuitive that malfunctions become less and less likely to mimic the pattern of activity that would be produced by a real sound, at progressively higher stations in the auditory system.

Similar restrictions may in fact occur at more peripheral levels because of the characteristic properties of neural phase-locking. This would mean that within the same (lower) frequency region, many fibres would have their neural firings synchronised by the auditory stimulus. It is possible that the high level of intolerance for, or discomfort felt with, certain forms of tinnitus, which by a matching technique might not be far above threshold, may be due to its unnatural behaviour in which firing *rate* may signal a stimulus, whereas correlation between firing *times* does not. It is interesting to note, however, that most tonal tinnitus matches are to higher frequencies where phase locking would not occur.

An entirely contrary approach is taken in a recent model proposed by Moller (1984) in which tinnitus might be due to the compression or destruction of the myelin sheath, allowing 'cross-talk' between fibres. The basis of this explanation is that the time of neural firings becomes synchronised, not to a stimulus, but to each other's spontaneous activity by ephaptic transmission. As Moller points out, there is a difficulty at high frequencies where phase-locking does not occur. Although it is possible that the brain might interpret synchrony of high-frequency fibres also as sound, the model becomes less plausible. The responses will, however, normally be correlated for high-frequency broad-band sounds, because of signal envelope information.

Another aspect of central processing concerns the role that efferent activity might play. If, for example, efferent activity exerts a non-specific inhibitory influence, set by the overall level of afferent activity, a restricted population of afferent activity might receive less inhibition than appropriate, leading to the false perception of sound within this region.

Otoacoustic emissions

Returning now to the periphery we consider the phenomena of OAEs and their relation to tinnitus. As mentioned earlier, OAEs were first looked for by Gold (1948) but not found until 1978 by Kemp. The general properties of OAEs will first be described. If a sound is introduced into the sealed ear canal, evidence for a delayed, non-linear, and frequency-filtered re-emission of sound can be obtained. An acoustic click will elicit a quite specific 'echo', characteristic of that particular ear, normally a short train of waves (Fig. 2.6). Continuous stimulation by a sine wave will lead to a continuous re-emission of sound at that frequency, observable as peaks and dips in the frequency-response curve due to interference with the stimulus (Fig. 2.7). The response behaves non-linearly because it does not increase in proportion to the stimulus, the waveshape of the response is level-dependent, suggesting a different input/output function for different frequencies and different time delays, and non-linear intermodulation components can be detected such as the frequency, $2f_1-f_2$, in response to the presented frequencies f_1 and f_2. In most cases the maximum level of re-emission seems to be limited to about 20 dB SPL (but see below). Thus if a typical acoustic measurement range of say 60–100 dB SPL is considered, the emitted sound represents a very small element. This feature probably accounts for the long time that it has taken for the phenomenon to be discovered. If, however, a low sound level is used with a good subject, and the frequency of stimulation is tuned to the subject's natural frequency of re-emission, which in turn is close to the resonance frequency of the middle ear, the re-emission can be less than 2 dB below the stimulus (Wilson 1980a). When we consider the inevitable losses inwards and outwards through the middle ear, this means that the acoustic signal must have been amplified within the inner ear. This is the same conclusion as reached above in connection with the recent very sharp and sensitive BM responses.

THEORY 33

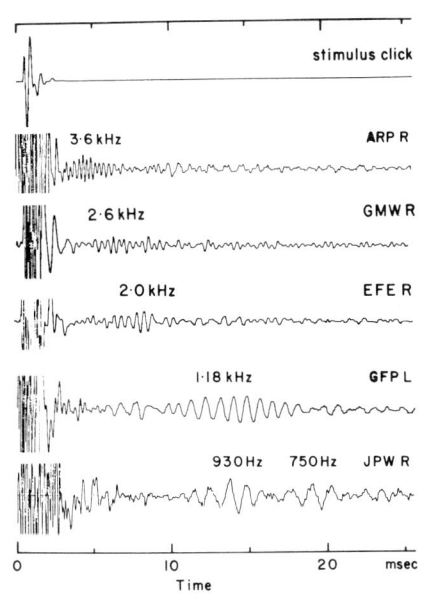

Fig. 2.6 Click-evoked OAEs from five human ears. The lower curves are amplified relative to the upper one, so that the first 3 ms represents stimulus overload. Note that OAEs of lower frequency have longer latency-to-peak response (from Wilson 1980b).

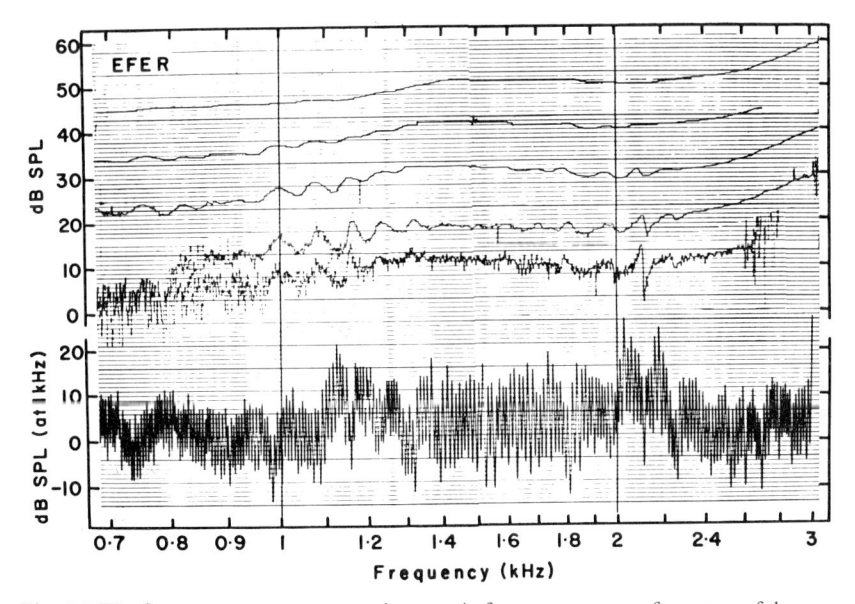

Fig. 2.7 The five upper curves represent the acoustic frequency response for system of the condenser-microphone driver, ear canal and electret microphone, at constant driver voltages in 10 dB steps. At the lower levels, ripples become progressively more prominent as re-emitted sound at the stimulus frequency interferes with the stimulus. Corresponding ripples can be seen in the Békésy-audiogram (bottom curve). At two positions SOAEs can be detected, and observed by the subject as tinnitus (from Wilson 1980b).

At the lowest sound levels the system behaves more linearly and, unlike neural responses, appears to have no threshold (Wilson 1980a). Evidence for continuous re-emission has been found down to −50 dB SPL, far below neural threshold (~ 0 dB SPL). It does, therefore, appear to depend on a quite different active process from that involved in neural spike initiation and conduction.

In general terms the frequency-filtering properties of the OAE suggest that the active process either follows, or is intimately associated with, the frequency-filtering properties of the cochlea. Strong evidence for this can be found in the sensitivity of the response to suppression by a second stimulus (Kemp & Chum 1980, Wilson 1980b, Zurek 1981). The tuning curves for this show a strong quantitative and qualitative resemblance to curves obtained psychophysically or by single unit recording (but see below).

One effect of interference between stimulus and re-emission is that the sensitivity of the ear, or audiogram, might be expected to be influenced in a related way. This had been found earlier by Elliott (1958) and Thomas (1975) and has been shown to be related to OAEs (Kemp 1979, Wilson 1980b, Zwicker & Schloth 1984). Even when a free-field earphone is used (Wilson 1980b), interference takes place due to internal reflection from the stapes footplate. The fine structure can be observed either as loudness enhancements for signals above threshold or as a series of fairly regularly spaced maxima and minima in the audiogram. It should be emphasised that the very narrow band-widths of individual peaks are a direct result of multiple internal reflection with a relatively long loop delay and should not be thought of as necessarily indicating very sharp independent filters as Manley (1983) suggests. This view is supported by the way peaks and dips can be caused to interchange by pressure on the middle ear (Wilson 1980b, Wilson & Sutton 1981). A single region of reflection within the cochlea is seen as being responsible for a group of maxima and minima with uniform spacing. There then may be a gap and then another group with a different spacing, which is greater for higher frequencies. On average, maxima may be logarithmically spaced (Kemp 1979, Zwicker & Schloth 1984) but within a group they tend to be equal (Wilson 1980b).

This feature of acoustic re-emission from certain places within the cochlea and not from others is a basic but incompletely understood property. It cannot simply represent regions where the active mechanisms are more strongly represented because that would imply that such frequency regions should have systematically lower thresholds, which they do not (Wilson 1980b). Kemp (1978, 1979) and Kim et al (1980) have suggested a reflection of the BM travelling wave by an impedance discontinuity whereas Wilson (1980c) and Sutton & Wilson (1983) have suggested that it is due to an irregularity in the frequency/place map. (For a more detailed discussion see Wilson 1984a.)

There is now much evidence that any factor that influences hearing also appears to influence the OAE. Such factors include short-term masking effects (Kemp 1981, Zwicker & Manley 1981, Zwicker 1983), longer-term (TTS) effects (Kemp 1981, Wilson & Evans 1983b), hypoxia (Evans et al 1981), drugs such as ethacrynic acid (Anderson & Kemp 1979) furosemide (Wilson & Evans 1983b), salicylates (Johnsen & Elberling 1982, McFadden & Plattsmier 1984).

Spontaneous otoacoustic emissions (SOAEs)

So far we have been considering evoked or continuously stimulated OAEs. When there is sufficient acoustic amplification for the internal reflection from the middle ear back into the cochlea to exceed the initial input, the signal level will build up and continuous oscillation result. Because the input/output function is non-linear, as the oscillation increases, the gain will decrease. This will stabilise the level to that at which the gain is unity. This accounts for the relatively modest level at which SOAEs usually occur (~ 0-20 dB SPL). At these low levels, internal noise has a considerable influence on the form and band-width of the oscillations (Kemp 1981). Quite modest levels of external signal, either clicks or continuous tones, can influence the spontaneous signal either by synchronising its phase (Wilson 1980b, Wilson & Sutton 1981) or shifting its frequency (Wilson & Sutton 1981) or indeed suppressing it (Kemp & Chum 1980, Wilson & Sutton 1981, Zurek 1981, Zwicker 1983).

SOAEs can also be influenced in a number of other ways, as for stimulated OAEs, including TTS (Kemp 1981) and hypoxia (Evans et al 1981), and by the effects of external ear pressure (Kemp 1979, Wilson & Sutton 1981). Attempts to demonstrate an influence of body temperature on SOAE frequency have not been convincing (Zurek 1981, Wilson 1984b, 1985) although there may be a slight periodic change of frequency throughout the menstrual cycle.

The audibility of SOAEs as tinnitus now seems to be fairly well established (see below). In general SOAEs do not appear to be related to the more distressing forms of tinnitus. In two cases in which particularly strong SOAEs had been recorded, subjects were initially not, and subsequently only marginally, aware of their own sounds (Wilson & Sutton 1983). In several cases, discovery of SOAEs and subsequent replay to the subject, has made them aware of their noises for the first (but not the last!) time.

An exception to the above pattern, however, is a subject who had a relatively severe high-frequency tinnitus located 'in the head'. Upon investigation (in collaboration with G. J. Sutton), it transpired that there were components in both ears sufficiently close in frequency to give a central fused image. This subject was unusual in two other respects, with a hearing loss at all frequencies except the tinnitus region (6–10 kHz) and in showing evidence for quite strong stimulated emissions at these high frequencies where the efficiency of the middle ear is believed to be low. This would appear to be evidence for the hypothesis that OAEs may be produced or enhanced by being on the borderline of a pathological region (Wilson & Sutton 1981, Sutton & Wilson 1983, Zurek & Clark 1981, Ruggero et al 1983).

It was also interesting to be able to follow up the cases of a brother and sister first reported by Glanville et al (1971) in which sound levels of up to 60 dB SPL had been measured at the entrance to the ear canal. More extensive later measurements revealed a very wide range of frequency components from 5.6 to 14 kHz at levels from −5 to +35 dB SPL. The follow-up (Wilson & Sutton 1983) revealed component levels up to 45 dB SPL, and the fact that various properties such as suppression by an external tone, and its influence in changing the emission frequency, were similar to those found for SOAEs. A somewhat discordant finding was that in two of the four ears concerned there was a quite substantial elevation of hearing threshold in the frequency range of SOAE components. This could be due to the masking effect of these very intense objective tones but this interpretation is compromised by their low audibility. The subjects initially reported that they were unaware of their own tones but after a considerable period of psychoacoustical testing in a sound-proofed room, they reversed this decision. Adaptation to a steady state does not appear to be a plausible explanation because their SOAE spectra showed frequent rapid changes (Fig. 1.8). In spite of this, however, there appeared to be a considerable correlation between the spectra obtained at the ages of 4 years and 4 months, respectively, with those obtained 13 years later at the ages of 17 years and 13 years. There was some indication that the main components might have shifted downwards by about 1%, presumably less than expected from cochlear growth changes. Remarkable also was the stability of the audiogram abnormalities mentioned above. If the audiogram loss is produced by hair-cell pathology, it does not appear to be progressive.

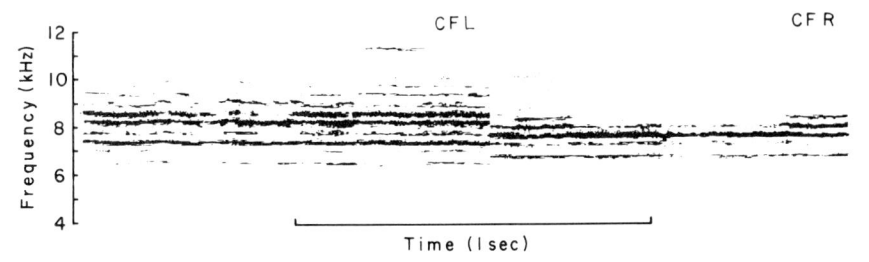

Fig. 2.8 Sonograms of two particularly strong SOAEs. Note how the spectral composition (dark bands) changes somewhat, quite rapidly, with time.

Comparative aspects of OAEs

Attempts to measure OAEs in different species have led to varying degrees of success. Such studies can lead to much greater understanding of the processes involved. Stimulus frequency emissions in man and monkey (Anderson & Kemp 1979) are generally stronger than responses in the cat (Wilson 1980c, Wilson & Evans 1983b) the guinea pig (Evans et al 1981, Zwicker & Manley 1981) the chinchilla (Zurek & Clark 1981) or the gerbil (Kemp & Brown 1983). This may be partly due to the shorter latencies involved and therefore the greater difficulty in separating the OAE from the middle-ear reflection and ringing (Wilson & Evans 1983b, Zwicker & Manley 1981). The shorter latency would imply less sharp filtering and this might in turn lead to greater uniformity of mapping along the cochlear partition, and therefore less OAE produced.

On the other hand, the above non-primates all appear to generate the intermodulation component $2f_1-f_2$ in greater proportions than man (Kim et al 1980, Kemp & Brown 1983, Wilson 1980d). Kemp & Brown (1983) found two components at $2f_1-f_2$ with different latencies. It appears that the shorter latency component might be independent of the signal frequency OAE mechanism.

OAEs have also been found in the caiman alligator (Strack et al 1981, see also Wilson 1984a, and Wilson et al 1985). This is surprising because it would seem that the frequency selective mechanism may be somewhat different in this species because its neural tuning is strongly temperature-dependent (Klinke & Smolders 1977, Smolers & Klinke 1984). Even more surprising is the finding of OAEs and SOAEs in the frog (Palmer & Wilson 1982) because in this species the hair cells are fixed and there is no analogue of the BM. Although it might be postulated that a travelling wave occurs in the overlying tectorial membrane, this cannot be a universal 'second-filter' mechanism because in the basal region of the basilar papilla of the alligator lizard there is no tectorial membrane and the BM is untuned although single neurones are nevertheless sharply tuned (Weiss et al 1978). The range of re-emission frequencies in the frog (0.5–2 kHz) would definitely appear to implicate the amphibian papilla, which is another temperature-sensitive hearing organ (Moffat & Capranica 1976), and possibly also the basilar papilla which is not. One possible implication of the finding of OAEs from such a wide range of animals is that it is a very general property of hair cells rather than a by-product of one specific type of active mechanical process. This has been the basis of one type of model for OAEs in which the synchronous swelling and shrinking of hair cells is postulated (Wilson 1980c) and receives possible support in the findings of Brownell et al (1985) who showed that isolated guinea pig outer hair cells change their length with electrical stimulation. In the latter case, however, it is possible that the length changes observed might be exactly counteracted by diameter changes.

In addition to the species specifically mentioned above (man, frog) SOAEs have also been found in the guinea pig (Evans et al 1981), the chinchilla (Zurek & Clark 1981) and the dog (Ruggero et al 1983). There have also been anecdotal reports of tonal emissions from the ears of a cat, a pony, and other dogs. The guinea-pig response is interesting because it was possible to demonstrate that some factors influenced it whereas others did not. It could be suppressed most strongly by an external tone around the SOAE frequency but also by a range of frequencies about three times higher. Similar remote effects of suppressions have also been found in man (Sutton 1985). Zurek (1981) reports a possibly related irregularity in the suppression curve, but the mechanism is not yet understood. It was also possible to follow the time course of suppression and release from suppression in the guinea pig and observe that it was identical for both the acoustic and round-window-electrical responses with a latency of about 4 ms. This is evidence that the OAE is not delayed by a reverse travelling wave relative to the electrical response (Wilson 1980c). Inducing middle-ear pressure attenuated the acoustic signal but not the electrical one, although a slight increase in frequency was noted. As expected, paralysis and later sectioning of the middle-ear muscles did not eliminate the SOAE whereas hypoxia reversibly abolished it.

In the chinchilla, Zurek & Clark (1981) were able to demonstrate SOAEs in two ears after a 0.5 kHz octave-band noise over-stimulatoin. In one of these no SOAE had been present before stimulation nor immediately afterwards, but had developed within 12 days. It was intially at 4.6 kHz but changed to 5.7 kHz from time to time. It could be suppressed readily by a tone in the same frequency region. In the other animal a tone of 6.4–6.7 kHz was observed which could beat with or be suppressed by an external tone. Behavioural audiograms before and after noise stimulation revealed that only at 6.7 kHz had the threshold fully recovered. Subsequent histology revealed a sharply localised destruction of all hair cells at the 7 kHz place. This again is support for the hypothesis that the border between normal and pathological hearing may be particularly susceptible to the generation of OAEs. Other similar lesions in this and other exposed animals were also found, so that the presence of such a lesion is not the only requirement for the generation of an SOAE. Nor, of course, can we be sure that the noise or the lesion actually caused the SOAE, or that the animals concerned perceived tinnitus.

TINNITUS IN HUMANS

Even before the SOAE was discovered attempts had been made to equate tinnitus with an active mechanical process (Gold 1948). The results attributing tinnitus to SOAEs have been variable but ultimately disappointing. Wilson (1980b) reported that in a survey of 40 ears, 10 produced SOAEs of which 7 were, after prompting, audible as tinnitus. Tyler & Conrad-Armes (1982) investigated 30 patients with sensorineural tinnitus and could find only one SOAE, which was unheard. Zurek (1981) reported that out of 32 normal-hearing subjects, SOAEs were detected in 22 ears from 16 of the subjects. None of the subjects was aware of tinnitus before the measurement although at least one was afterwards. On the other hand, six subjects who claimed to have tinnitus produced no corresponding SOAE. Wilson & Sutton (1981) reported further on some of the subjects mentioned above (Wilson 1980b) and included a further group of six subjects who would be described as tinnitus sufferers. Two of the latter had SOAEs, one unheard, the other, although audible, was not the predominant tinnitus component. In all members of this group, tinnitus appeared to be localised in a region of audiogram deficit. One of this group (ITM) was recently reinvestigated and surprisingly both the audiogram notches and the tinnitus had shifted upwards from 6–7 kHz to 9 kHz. Rabinowitz & Widkin (1984) found SOAEs in 8 ears out of 19 tested from 12 normal-hearing subjects. Only one subject perceived tinnitus. Schloth (1983) found SOAEs in 22 out of 64 normal ears. In a later study (Wilson & Sutton, unpublished) of about 60 tinnitus sufferers only one had corresponding SOAEs (see above) and one had unheard SOAEs. Again, in most cases tinnitus comes from a region of audiogram deficit although not necessarily the region of greatest loss. In many cases it was in a region of rapid change of slope.

The general conclusions are that SOAEs occur in a high proportion of normal ears (about one-third) and do not generally give rise to complaints of tinnitus whereas clinically-reported tinnitus is rarely due to SOAEs and is frequently associated with hearing loss. Kemp (1981) has pointed out, however, that cochlear mechanical vibration could conceivably occur on a local scale at too low a level to be detected. This would be particularly likely if, as Tonndorf (1980) suggested, pathology and hearing loss result from a decoupling of the receptor from the tectorial membrane. At this stage, however, it has to be accepted as more likely that sensorineural tinnitus is generated beyond the mechanical stage. One piece of evidence supporting this view is that most attempts at obtaining beats with this type of tinnitus have failed (McFadden 1982).

There are in fact a number of ways in which tinnitus does not behave like a normal external sound (McFadden 1982):

1. Frequencies remote from the tinnitus match can sometimes mask it (Feldman 1971, 1981, Vernon & Meikle 1981).
2. Masking levels may be much greater or much less than expected for an external signal, or the tinnitus may be unmaskable.
3. The masking level may 'adapt' with time, requiring 30–45 dB more after half an hour of masking (Penner et al 1981).
4. Contralateral masking frequently occurs (Feldman 1971, 1981) at about the same level as that required for ipsilateral masking.
5. Residual inhibition can last from seconds to several hours after termination of the masker (Feldman 1971, 1981).
6. A similar tinnitus in both ears will often not fuse but remain localized at the ears (Vernon 1978).

Some of these factors (1–4) seem intuitively reasonable if the source of tinnitus is located more centrally, but factors 5 and 6 are difficult to explain.

ANIMAL MODELS OF TINNITUS

Although it would be difficult to devise a behavioural test for animal perception of tinnitus, it seems reasonable to assume that influences that induce tinnitus in man may also do so in animals. Animal models for SOAE-related tinnitus have already been discussed above. This section will consider possible correlates of tinnitus where this is associated with hearing loss caused by noise overdose, hydrops and drugs such as salicylate, quinine, loop diuretics, aminoglycocides, etc.

Kiang et al (1970) reported on kanamycin-induced hearing loss in the cat. Hair cells in the basal region were found to be missing (19–136 days following the last dose). No responses from high-frequency stimulation were found, although lower-frequency regions remained intact. Many units had zero or very low spontaneous activity and could be stimulated only electrically. They postulate that tinnitus either arises from *absence* of activity or from the abnormal spatial pattern of activity, the *border* between a normal and pathological region being a particularly strong candidate.

Liberman & Kiang (1978), also working with cats, found that after intense noise-band stimulation, spontaneous rates were reduced in regions where the sensistivity to sound was reduced. Salvi et al (1978) found a similar result for chinchilla cochlear nucleus neurones.

Schmiedt et al (1980) using gerbils found a similar result to Kiang et al (1970) for kanamycin, but the opposite effect to Liberman & Kiang (1978) and Salvi et al (1978), for noise exposure. Dallos and Harris (1978) failed to find a change in spontaneous rate for chinchillas after kanamycin. Most other studies tend to find a reduction of spontaneous rate with acute pathology (see Evans 1975).

Evans et al (1981) gave cats large divided doses of sodium salicylate. The single fibre thresholds were found to go up for all CFs (although rather more so for higher CFs) in line with human audiogram findings (Myers & Bernstein 1965, Mongan et al

1973). But contrary to most of the studies mentioned above, the mean spontaneous rate, for the higher rate fibres at least, was found to increase slightly (from 59 to 78 spikes/s). As this occurred over all CFs, no edge effect could be involved. Furthermore it appears that in most cases, salicylate-induced tinnitus has a high-pitched rather than a broad-band nature.

Another interesting finding from this study was that some spontaneous spikes appeared to occur in pairs giving a bimodal interspike interval histogram (Fig. 2.9). This effect has only been observed previously for noise-driven activity and suggests that the brain might interpret it as such. An intravenous injection of lignocaine was followed by a slight reduction of spontaneous activity, but this was too small to be considered significant.

Prijs & Harrison (1984) studied an animal model of endolymphatic hydrops in two guinea pigs. Microdissection afterwards confirmed the hydrops but found no

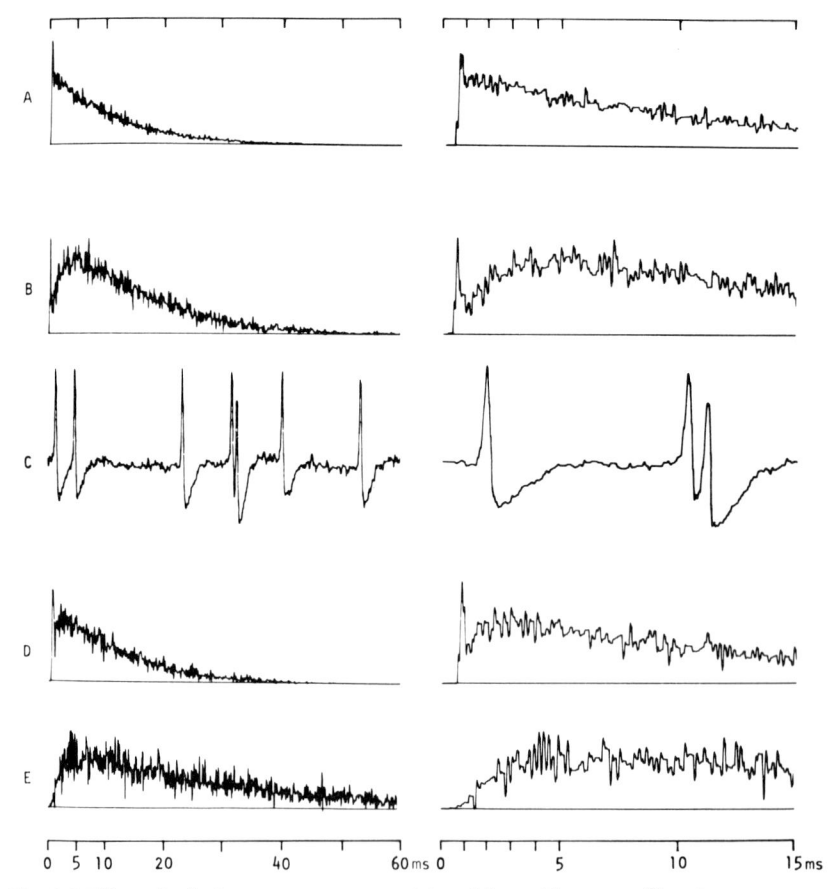

Fig. 2.9 Effects of salicylate on spontaneous activity of the cochlear nerve fibre shows on two different time scales (left and right). (C) shows the anomalous occurrence of paired spikes. The effects of this on the interspike interval histogram are shown in (A and B) compared with a normal fibre (E). A similar effect is produced in (D) by stimulation with broadband noise 50 dB above threshold (from Evans et al 1981). By permission of Pitman Publishing Ltd., London

evidence of hair cell damage. CAP audiograms were raised by about 40 dB in both animals. Single fibre thresholds were similarly increased and their Q_{10dB} values reduced. Five percent of units showed spontaneous bursting activity which the authors suggest might be related to tinnitus. It should be noted, however, that endolymphatic hydrops is not an adequate model for Ménière's syndrome (Schuknecht 1984).

GENERAL CONCLUSIONS

The above reports show promising results for animal models although these clearly need to be extended. Certain aspects of SOAE-related tinnitus are now understood although the underlying active mechanical process has not yet been identified. This, however, seems to be a relatively innocuous form of tinnitus. It is considered possible, but unlikely, that other forms of tinnitus may also be related to mechanical activity if the hair cell becomes decoupled from the input. Many forms of tinnitus are associated with audiogram abnormalities caused by presbyacusis, noise exposure, viral infection, drug damage, etc. If this is due to an abnormal pattern of spontaneous neural firing it raises some problems. Why are not all irregularities in the audiogram associated with tinnitus? Why are certain drugs such as lignocaine effective in many such cases, when it is unlikely that they could alter the abnormality of the pattern in any significant way? Does the influence of melanin hold some clues (Lyttkens et al 1978)? Why does tinnitus sometimes occur in the absence of any hearing loss, with drugs, and pathologies such as Ménières disease, that produce a flat hearing loss? Although the neural bursting activity discussed above (Evans et al 1981, Prijs & Harrison 1984) might be one explanation, theories for tinnitus generation are still largely speculative. This unfortunately appears to be even more so for more central forms of tinnitus where a wide variety of different behaviour is found.

REFERENCES

Aitkin L M, Webster W R 1984 In: Handbook of Physiology, Am Physiol Soc. Williams and Wilkins, Baltimore

Anderson S D, Kemp D T 1979 The evoked cochlear mechanical response in laboratory primates, a preliminary report. Archives of Otorhinolaryngology 224: 47–54

Békésy G von 1953 Journal of the Acoustic Society of America 25: 770–785

Békésy G von 1960 Experiments in hearing. McGraw Hill, New York

Brownell W E, Bader C R, Bertrand D, Ribaupierre Y de 1985 Evoked mechanical response in isolated cochlear outer hair cells. Science 227: 194–196

Cazals Y, Negrevergne M, Aran J-M 1978 Electrical stimulation of the cochlea in man: hearing induction and tinnitus suppression. Journal of the American Audiological Society 3: 209–213

Crawford A C, Fettiplace R 1981 An electrical tuning mechanism in turtle cochlear hair cells. Journal of Physiology 312: 377–412

Crosby E, Humphrey T, Lauer E 1962 Correlative anatomy of the nervous system. Macmillan, New York

Dallos P 1975 Cochlear potentials. In: The Nervous System (Ed) Tower D P, Vol 3: Human Communication and Its Disorders. Raven Press, New York

Dallos P 1985 Response characteristics of mammalian cochlear hair cells. Journal of Neuroscience 5: 1591–1608

Dallos P, Harris D 1978 Properties of auditory nerve responses in absence of outer hair cells. Journal of Neurophysiology 41: 365–383
de Boer E 1980 Auditory physics. Physical principles in hearing theory I. Physics Reports 62: 87–174
Elliott E 1958 A ripple effect in the audiogram. Nature 181: 1076
Evans E F 1972 Journal of Physiology 226: 263–287
Evans E F 1975 Cochlear nerve and cochlear nucleus. In: Handbook of sensory physiology. Keidel W D, Neff W D (eds), Vol V (2), Springer, Berlin
Evans E F, Wilson J P 1973 The frequency selectivity of the cochlea. In: Basic mechanisms in hearing. A R Møller (ed), Academic Press, New York, pp 519–554
Evans E F, Wilson J P 1975 Cochlear tuning properties—concurrent basilar membrane and single nerve fiber measurements. Science 190: 1218–1221
Evans E F, Wilson J P, Borerwe T A 1981 Animal models of tinnitus. In: Tinnitus. Evered D, Lawrenson G (eds) Ciba Foundation Symposium 85, Pitman, London, pp 108–138
Feldmann H 1971 Homolateral and contralateral masking of tinnitus by noise-bands and by pure tones. Audiology 10: 138–144
Feldmann H 1981 Homolateral and contralateral masking of tinnitus. Journal of Laryngology and Otology, Supplement 4: 60–70
Glanville J D, Coles R R A, Sullivan B M 1971 A family with high-tonal objective tinnitus. Journal of Laryngology and Otology 85: 1–10
Gold T 1948 Hearing II The physical basis of the action of the cochlea. Proceedings of the Royal Society B 135: 492–498
Johnsen N J, Elberling C 1982 Evoked acoustic emissions from the human ear. Scandinavian Audiology 11: 3–12
Johnstone B M 1983 Mechanics of the mammalian cohclea. Proceedings of the International Union of Physiological Sciences (Sydney) 15: 113.01
Johnstone B M, Taylor K J, Boyle A J 1970 Mechanics of the guinea pig cochlea. Journal of the Accoustical Society of America 47: 504–509
Kemp D T 1978 Stimulated acoustic emissions from within the human auditory system. Journal of the Acoustical Society of America 64: 1386–1391
Kemp D T 1979 The evoked cochlear mechanical response and the auditory microstructure: evidence for a new element in cochlear mechanics. Scandinavian Audiology Supplement 9: 35–47
Kemp D T 1981 Physiologically active cochlear micromechanics–one source of tinnitus. In: Tinnitus. Evered D, Lawrenson G (eds) Ciba Foundation Symposium 85, Pitman, London pp 54–81
Kemp D T, Brown A M 1983 A comparison of mechanical nonlinearities in the cochleae of man and gerbil from ear canal measurements. In: Hearing–physiological bases and psychophysics, Klinke R, Hartmann R (eds), Springer, Berlin, pp 82–88
Kemp D T, Chum R 1980 Properties of the generator of stimulated acoustic emissions. Hearing Research 2: 213–232
Khanna S M 1983 Interpretation of the sharply tuned basilar membrane response observed in the cochlea. In: Hearing and other senses: Presentations in honor of E G Wever. Fay R R, Gourevitch G (eds), Amphora Press, Groton CT, pp 65–86
Khanna S M, Leonard D G B 1982 Basilar membrane tuning in the cat cochlea. Science 215: 305–306
Kiang N Y S, Moxon E C, Levine R A 1970 Auditory-nerve activity in cats with normal and abnormal cochleas. In: Sensorineural hearing loss Wolstenholme G E W, Knight J (eds), Churchill, London, pp 241–273
Kiang N Y S, Watanabe T, Thomas E C, Clark L F 1965 Discharge patterns of single fibers in the cat's auditory nerve. Research Monograph 35, MIT Press, Cambridge, Mass.
Kim D O, Neely S T, Molnar C E, Matthews J W 1980 An active cochlear model with negative damping within the partition: comparison with Rhode's ante- and post-mortem observations. In: Psychophysical physiological and behavioural studies in hearing, van den Brink G, Bilsen F A (eds), Delft University Press, pp 7–14
Klinke R, Smolders J 1977 Effect of temperature shift on tuning properties. In: Psychophysics and physiology of hearing, Evans E F, Wilson J P (eds), Academic Press, London, pp 109–111
Klochoff I 1981 Impedance fluctuation and a 'tensor tympani' syndrome. In: Acoustic impedance measurements. Penha and Pizarro (eds.) University of Lisbon, pp 69–76
Liberman M C 1982 The cochlear frequency map for the cat: labeling auditory nerve fibers of known characteristic frequency. Journal of the Acoustical Society of America 72: 1441–1449

Liberman M C, Kiang N Y S 1978 Acoustic trauma in cats. Acta Otolaryngologica Supplement 358: 1–63
Lim D J 1980 Cochlear anatomy related to cochlear micromechanics. A review. Journal of the Acoustical Society of America 67: 1686–1695
Lyttkens L, Larsson B, Stahle J, Englesson S 1979 Accumulation of substances with melanin affinity to the internal ear. Advances in Oto-Rhino-Laryngology 25: 17–25
McFadden D 1982 Tinnitus: Facts, theories, and treatments. National Academy Press, Washington DC
McFadden D, Plattsmier H S 1984 Aspirin abolishes spontaneous oto-acoustic emissions. Journal of the Acoustical Society of America 76: 443–448
Manley G A 1983 Frequency spacing of acoustic emissions: a possible explanation. In: Mechanisms of hearing, Webster W R, Aitkin L M (eds), Monash University Press, Clayton, Victoria, 36–39
Moffat A J M, Capranica R R 1976 Effects of temperature on the response properties of auditory nerve fibres in the American toad *Bufo americanus*. Journal of the Acoustical Society of America 60: Supplement 1, S80 (abstract)
Møller A R 1984 Pathophysiology of tinnitus. Annals of Otology Rhinology and Laryngology 93: 39–44
Mongan E, Kelly P, Nies K, Porter W W, Paulus H E 1973 Tinnitus as an indication of therapeutic serum salicylate levels. Journal of the American Medical Association 226: 142–145
Myers E N, Bernstein J M 1965 Salicylate ototoxicity: a clinical and experimental study. Archives of Otolaryngology 82: 483–493
O'Connor A F, Shea J J 1981 Autophony and the patulous Eustachian tube. Laryngoscope 91. 1427–1435
Palmer A R, Wilson J P 1982 Spontaneous and evoked acoustic emissions in the frog *Rana esculenta*. Journal of Physiology 324: 66P
Penner M J, Brauth S, Hood L 1981 The temporal course of the masking of tinnitus as a basis for inferring its origin. Journal of Speech and Hearing Research 24: 257–261
Prijs V P, Harrison R V 1984 Eighth nerve responses in guinea pigs with long term endolymphatic hydrops. Revue de Laryngologie-Otologie-Rhinologie 105: Supplement 2, 229–235
Rabinowitz W M, Widkin G P 1984 Interaction of spontaneous oto-acoustic emissions and external sounds. Journal of the Acoustical Society of America 76: 1713–1720
Rhode W S 1971 Observations of the vibration of the basilar membrane in squirrel monkeys using the Mossbauer technique. Journal of the Acoustical Society of America 49: 1218–1231
Rhode W S 1978 Some observations on cochlear mechanics. Journal of the Acoustical Society of America 64: 158–176
Robertson D, Manley G A 1974 Manipulation of frequency analysis in the cochlear ganglion of the guinea pig. Journal of Comparative Physiology 91: 363–375
Ruggero M A, Rich N C, Freyman R 1983 Spontaneous and impulsively evoked otoacoustic emissions: indicators of cochlear pathology? Hearing Research 10: 283–300
Russell I J, Sellick P M 1978 Intracellular studies of hair cells in the mammalian cochlea. Journal of Physiology 284: 261–290
Salvi R J, Hamernik R P, Handerson D 1978 Discharge patterns in the cochlear nucleus of the chinchilla following noise-induced asymptotic threshold shift. Experimental Brain Research 32: 301–320
Schloth E 1983 Relation between spectral composition of spontaneous oto-acoustic emissions and fine structure of threshold in quiet. Acustica 53: 250–256
Schmiedt R A, Zwislocki J J, Hamernik R P 1980 Effects of hair cell lesions on responses of cochlear nerve fibers. Journal of Neurophysiology 43: 1367–1389
Schuknecht H F 1984 Histopathology of the ear and its clinical implications. Symposium in honour of Harold F Schuknecht. Annals of Otology, Rhinology and Laryngology Supplement. Nadol J B & Wilson W R (eds)
Sellick, P M, Patuzzi R, Johnstone B M 1982 Measurement of basilar membrane motion in the guinea pig using the Mössbauer technique. Journal of the Acoustical Society of America 72: 131–141
Smolders J, Klinke R 1984 Effects of temperature on the properties of primary auditory fibres of the spectacled caiman, *Caiman crocodilus* (L.). Journal of Comparative Physiology 155: 19–30
Spoendlin H 1967 The innervation of the organ of Corti. Jounral of Laryngology and Otology 81: 717–738
Strack G, Klinke R, Wilson J P 1981 Evoked cochlear response in *Caiman crocodilus*. Pfluger's Archives Supplement 391: R43

Suga N, Neuweiler G, Moller J 1976 Peripheral auditory tuning for fine frequency analysis by the CF-FM bat, *Rhinolophus ferrumequinum*. IV. Properties of peripheral auditory neurons. Journal of Comparative Physiology 106: 111–125

Sutton G J, 1985 Suppression effects in the spectrum of evoked otoacoustic emissions. Acoustica 58: 57–63

Sutton G J, Wilson J P 1983 Modelling cochlear echoes: the influence of irregularities in frequency mapping on summed cochlear activity. In: Mechanisms of hearing, Boer E de, Viergever M A (eds) Delft University Press, pp 1183–1192

Thomas I B 1975 Microstructure of the pure tone threshold. Journal of the Acoustical Society of America 57, Supplement 1: S26–S27 (abstract)

Tonndorf J 1966 Bone conduction: studies in experimental animals. Acta Otolaryngologica, Supplement 213

Tonndorf J 1980 Acute cochlear disorders; the combination of hearing loss, recruitment, poor speech discrimination, and tinnitus. Annals of Otology Rhinology and Laryngology 89: 353–358

Tonndorf J, Khanna S M 1970 The role of the tympanic membrane in middle ear transmission. Annals of Otology Rhinology and Laryngology 79: 743–753

Tyler R S, Conrad-Armes D 1982 Spontaneous acoustic cochlear emissions and sensorineural tinnitus. British Journal of Audiology 16: 193–194

Vernon J 1978 Information from UOHSC tinnitus clinic. American Tinnitus Association Newsletter 3: 1–4

Vernon J, Meikle M B 1981 Tinnitus masking: unresolved problems. In: Tinnitus, CIBA Foundation Symposium 85, Evered D, Lawrenson G (eds), Pitman, London, pp 239–256

Walford R E 1983 A classification of environmental 'hums' and low frequency tinnitus. Journal of Low Frequency Noise and Vibration 2: 60–84

Weiss T F, Peake W T, Ling A, Holton T 1978 Which structures determine frequency selectivity and tonotopic organisation of vertibrate cochlear nerve fibres? In: Evoked electrical activity in the auditory nervous system. Naunton R, Fernandez C (eds), Academic Press, New York, pp 9–112

Wever E G 1978 The reptile ear. Princeton University Press, New Jersey

Wilson J P 1980a Subthreshold mechanical activity within the cochlea. Journal of Physiology 298: 32–33P

Wilson J P 1980b Evidence for a cochlear origin for acoustic re-emissions threshold fine-structure and tonal tinnitus. Hearing Research 2: 233–252

Wilson J P 1980c Model for cochlear echoes and tinnitus based on an observed electrical correlate. Hearing Research 2: 527–532

Wilson J P 1980d The combination tone $2f_1-f_2$ in psychophysics and ear-canal recording. In: Psychophysical physiological and behavioural studies in hearing. van den Brink G, Bilsen F A (eds), Delft University Press, pp 43–52

Wilson J P 1984a Otoacoustic emissions and hearing mechanisms. Revue de Laryngologie-Otologie-Rhinologie 105 Supplement 2: 179-191

Wilson J P 1984b The influence of temperature and body cycles on spontaneous otoacoustic emission frequency. British Journal of Audiology 18: 256 (abstract)

Wilson J P 1985 The influence of temperature on frequency tuning mechanisms. Mechanics of Hearing Workshop, Boston

Wilson J P, Bruns V 1983 Basilar membrane tuning properties in the specialised cochlea of the CF-bat, *Rhinolophus ferrumequinum*. Hearing Research 10: 15–35

Wilson J P, Evans E F 1983a Some observations on the 'passive' mechanics of cat basilar membrane. In: Mechanisms of hearing, Webster W R, Aitkin L M (eds), Monash University Press, Clayton, Victoria, Australia, pp 30–35

Wilson J P, Evans E F 1983b Effects of furosemide, flaxedil, noise and tone-overstimulation on the evoked oto-acoustic emission in cat. Proceedings of the International Union of Physiological Sciences (Sydney) 15: 186.07

Wilson J P, Johnstone J R 1975 Basilar membrane and middle-ear vibration in guinea pig measured by capacitive probe. Journal of the Acoustical Society of America 57: 705–723

Wilson J P, Sutton G J 1981 Acoustic correlates of tonal tinnitus. In: Tinnitus. Ciba Foundation Symposium 85. Evered D, Lawrenson G (eds), Pitman, London, pp 82–101

Wilson J P, Sutton G J 1983 'A family with high tonal objective tinnitus'—an update. In: Hearing–physiological bases and and psychophysics. Klinke R, Hartmann R (eds), Springer, Berlin, pp 79–84

Wilson J P, Smolders J W T, Klinke R 1985 Mechanics of the basilar membrane in *Caiman crocodilus*. Hearing Research 18: 1–14

Zurek P M 1981 Spontaneous narrowband acoustic signals emitted by human ears. Journal of the Acoustical Society of America 69: 514–523

Zurek P M, Clark W W 1981 Narrow-band acoustic signals emitted by chinchilla ears after noise exposure. Journal of the Acoustical Society of America 70: 446–450

Zwicker E 1983 On peripheral processing in human hearing. In: Hearing–physiological bases and psychophysics, Klinke R, Hartmann R (eds), Springer, Berlin, pp 104–110

Zwicker E, Manley G A 1981 Acoustical responses and suppression-period patterns in guinea pigs. Hearing Research 4: 43–52

Zwicker E, Schloth E 1984 Interrelation of different oto-acoustic emissions. Journal of the Acoustical Society of America 75: 1148–1154

3   *MRC Institute of Hearing Research*

Epidemiology of tinnitus

PREVALENCE OF TINNITUS

In recent years, there have been two large-scale population studies of tinnitus, both in the UK. The first is the National Study of Hearing (NSH) which is being conducted by the Medical Research Council's Institute of Hearing Research (IHR) from its headquarters in Nottingham and its clinical outstations in Cardiff, Glasgow, Nottingham and Southampton. This started in 1978 and is now in its third phase. The second study was part of the General Household Survey carried out in 1981 by the UK Office of Population Censuses and Surveys (OPCS). The rationale and methodology of the NSH and the tinnitus prevalence data obtained up to the time of writing, together with those from the OPCS survey, will form the basis of the prevalence section of this chapter.

National Study of Hearing

The NSH is a multi-purpose study of normal hearing and hearing disorders (including tinnitus) in the population covering the domains of pathology and possible pathological influences, impairment, disability and to a lesser extent handicap. Its many purposes have been described elsewhere (Institute of Hearing Research 1981a) but include obtaining the prevalence data needed for planning of clinical services and further research, and also control data for other studies allowing matching of variables such as age, gender, noise exposure and socio-economic group which the study itself has shown to be important. The influence of these and other variables on prevalence of hearing impairment and tinnitus in the population is now being studied in further detail (in Phase III), and in a longitudinal sequel from which it is hoped that further information on the determinants of hearing impairment and tinnitus may be identified.

    The basic plan of the study has been described elsewhere (Institute of Hearing Research 1981a,b, Coles 1984a) and need not be repeated here. The initial sampling (Tier A) was at random from the electoral registers of the four cities in which the IHR has its outstations. The postal questionnaire was short and simple, to produce high

---

This chapter was prepared by R R A Coles in collaboration with A C Davis and M P Haggard. The data analyses were carried out specifically for this chapter by Helen Spencer.

response rates (81%, after up to two reminders). It enabled the respondents to be stratified by self-reported hearing state (no complaint, hearing disorder, tinnitus, or hearing disorder plus tinnitus), age, gender, occupational noise exposure, and hearing-aid possession. Quotas were then sampled in each stratum. This double sampling greatly improved the efficiency of the subsequent prevalence estimates of hearing levels or other data obtained in the more intensive in-clinic investigations (Tier B) by comparison with ordinary random sampling. A telephone follow-up of a proportion of the remaining non-responders was made to check on possible biases, which were found to be quite small.

The acceptance rate of those subsequently invited to come into the clinic was about 50%. Domiciliary follow-up, including simple audiometry, was carried out to check on possible biases in the non-accepters. Again, these biases were minimal, apart from a suspected low compliance rate from ethnic-minority immigrants, on the size and effect of which it has proven very difficult to obtain quantitative information.

In the clinic (Tier B), an otological examination was performed together with a detailed clinical history of otological and general physical disorders, drugs taken, and other possible aetiological factors past and present. In the first two phases, blood samples were taken for haematology, general blood chemistry, liver, thyroid and renal function tests, and syphilis serology. Throughout, conventional audiometric tests were carried out including tympanometry and acoustic reflex measurements. The core of medical and audiometric assessment was supplemented by a range of further tests, which varied from phase to phase but typically included tests of frequency resolution and of audio-visual speech communication ability, together with specific conditional tests, notably those on tinnitus (when present).

The prevalence figures for different degrees of tinnitus cover a wide range, and it is therefore critically important to note: 1. the exact working of the questions asked; 2. the response alternatives; and 3. the manner in which the questionnaires were administered. Therefore, the tinnitus questions and response alternatives in the Tier A postal questionnaires are given in Appendix 3.1 at the end of this chapter. There is no single condition of 'tinnitus' that can be given a fixed definition and a single prevalence figure. Instead, there is a series of figures depending on the descriptions of the severity of the tinnitus.

Further generalisation beyond the outstation cities has been made possible by the Household Study, a component of the NSH. This was also conducted in two tiers, but based entirely on domiciliary visiting for Tier B. The sampling frame was households from the Post Office list of postal addresses in stratified electoral districts spread widely through the UK. One of its purposes was to ascertain the degree to which estimated prevalences for the four outstation cities may be applicable to the whole population, including those living in rural areas. As even double sampling cannot conveniently assess rare conditions, the Severe Deafness Study, another component of the NSH, is currently enumerating the prevalence of total and severe deafness and associated tinnitus in the population. This is being carried out in the Wessex Health Region (population about 2.5 million) by an inventory procedure going through all the relevant care agencies, e.g. general practitioners, otolaryngologists, social services staff.

Pilot Phase

Those with tinnitus of 'less than 5 minutes duration' and with tinnitus only experienced 'just after very loud sounds, e.g. discos, shooting, or noise at work', were excluded (see Appendix 3.1, Pilot Phase, introductory sentences). Those not so excluded are described here and subsequently as having spontaneous tinnitus of over 5 minutes duration. The prevalence of such ranged from 15.5% (Southampton) to 18.6% (Glasgow). Tinnitus causing moderate and severe degrees of annoyance was reported by about 4% and 1% respectively (Institute of Hearing Research 1981a,b). Interference with 'getting to sleep' was reported by about 5%. Tinnitus having a severe effect on 'ability to lead a normal life' was reported by about 0.5%

Cross-tabulations (Institute of Hearing Research 1981a) showed that only about four-fifths of those reporting moderate to severe annoyance from their tinnitus, or severe effects on their ability to lead a normal life, reported that tinnitus interfered with their getting to sleep. This has some importance as a warning to the clinician not to rely solely on a history of sleep disturbance as an indicator of severity of tinnitus, as appears to be a quite common practice. Likewise the severity of tinnitus is sometimes judged by whether it is present continuously or intermittently. The relationship between this aspect and tinnitus annoyance has also been studied (in Phase II, Tier B data), but absolutely no association was found. Thus, to judge the severity of tinnitus, a description is needed of a whole range of possible effects, e.g. the degree of annoyance it causes, its interference with speech communication, thinking and getting to sleep, and its effects on quality of life overall.

Phases I and II

The prevalences of tinnitus of varying degrees of severity as indicated by Phases I and II are shown in Table 3.1, together with comparative data from the Pre-Pilot and Pilot Phases. Tinnitus of unrestricted type and duration appears to have been experienced

Table 3.1 POPULATION PREVALENCES OF TINNITUS. Percentages of people reporting experience of various degrees of tinnitus in response to Tier A questionnaires in four phases of the National Study of Hearing. (Random samples from Cardiff, Glasgow, Nottingham and Southampton: combined data. After Coles, 1984a)

	Pre-Pilot	Pilot	Phase I	Phase II
n, valid data	522	5000	8069	7645
Tinnitus (any type)	39[1,2]	—	38.0[1]	33.8[1,3]
Tinnitus (<5[1] and/or non-spontaneous)	—	—	27.0	23.2
Difference (=spontaneous tinnitus >5[1])	—	—	11.0	−10.6
Tinn (spontaneous and >5[1])	—	17.5	—	—
Interference with getting to sleep	—	5.6	7.4	7.0
Moderate/severe annoyance	—	5.7	8.1	8.7
Severe effect on quality	—	—	—	1.0
Severe effect on ability	—	0.5	—	—

[1] Questions changed between phases with respect to when the tinnitus had been experienced, as follows: Pilot Study: 'Have you ever noticed . . . ?' Phase I: 'Do you ever get . . . ?' Phase II: 'Nowadays do you ever get . . . ?'
[2,3] Similar questions were asked in Phase III, giving prevalence rates in the 17 238 respondents of 46.7%[2] and 35.2%[3]: see section on natural history of tinnitus later in this chapter.

at some time by about 40% of the adult population. There were slight differences in the prevalence values derived from the Pilot Study and Phase I and Phase II. These could be accounted for by different wordings and arrangements of the questions asked. For an explanation of these the reader is referred to the original source (Coles 1984a).

A question on general effects on life was asked in the Pilot Phase, expressed in terms of 'affect your *ability* to lead a normal life' (question B3). In Phase II it was expressed in less severe terms, 'affect the *quality* of your life as a whole' (question B7). The corresponding prevalence rate shifted from 0.5% to 1% ($p=0.01$) with this change of wording, which was in the direction to be expected.

In a review of earlier American surveys, Leske (1981) quoted a prevalence of 'severe tinnitus' of 5.6%, which is supported now by the general pattern of prevalences for UK urban populations shown in Table 3.1. lying somewhere between the prevalences of moderate and severe annoyance. She also reported the results of a question about experience of tinnitus of any type or duration that has occurred 'at any time over the past few years'. This gave a prevalence of 32%, which is again in good agreement with the NSH data and also with the data of Hinchcliffe (1961).

General Household Survey

The GHS has been running continuously since 1971, collecting information by personal interview on a wide variety of topics for the use of various government departments. In 1981, a short series of questions on tinnitus was included at the request of the Department of Health and Social Security and responses to these were obtained from more than 23 000 persons aged 16 and over.

The report (Office of Population Censuses and Surveys 1983) on the prevalence of tinnitus stated: 'Overall, 22% of adults interviewed said that they had heard noises in their head or ears such as ringing or buzzing sounds. Subsequent questions established that in about one-third of these informants the noises were brought on only by an external stimulus—a loud noise, water getting in the ears, or colds and catarrh'. The wording of the questions with respect to severity was different from the NSH, but the most comparable group were probably those that said they were 'bothered a great deal' or 'bothered quite a lot'. Two percent of the population said 'Yes' to one or other of those questions. This is a lower figure than might have been expected from the NSH data, but the difference may be due to the fact that the OPCS study was done by personal interview, while the NSH study was based on postal questionnaires. On the other hand, the 5.6% 'severe tinnitus' figure quoted by Leske (1981) was also based on interviews; compared with the OPCS result, it may reflect a higher prevalence of troublesome tinnitus in the USA, or possibly a difference in the way in which peoples of different national culture respond to specific questions.

Prevalence: summary

To judge from the results of the Household Study, and also from information in early phases of the main study on how much of their life each subject had lived in urban or rural communities, there is reason to believe that the tinnitus prevalence data derived from the four NSH city samples are applicable to the country as a whole. In generalising to other countries, however, differences associated with climate, noise exposure of all types (occupational, military, leisure, domestic and community), socio-economic structure, race and diet have to be considered and may modify the prevalence rates. In spite of these uncertainties, some estimates of tinnitus prevalence in the adult (age 17 and over) populations of industrialised countries, are worthwhile, as follows:

> About 35–45% if adults appear to have experienced tinnitus of some type or duration at some time. While many of these are not what might be termed 'clinical tinnitus', even the non-spontaneous and short-duration ones appear to be a nuisance to some of these people (Coles 1984a).

> About 15% of adults appear to have or to have had spontaneous tinnitus lasting over 5 minutes.

> At least 8% experience tinnitus causing interference with their getting to sleep, and/or moderate or severe annoyance. This would suggest about 4 million adults in the UK being so affected.

> At the top end of the spectrum of severity come those 0.5% who report that their tinnitus has a severe effect on their ability to lead a normal life. As a percentage 0.5% sounds small, but this still amounts to about 200 000 persons in the UK. Moreover, tinnitus of this severity is at least comparable in terms of prevalence, of effects on health and quality of life, and of effectiveness of its treatment, to many other conditions of the ear. It therefore deserves much greater clinical attention than it has usually received up to now.

DETERMINANTS OF TINNITUS

Age and noise

In the pilot phase of the NSH (Institute of Hearing Research 1981a), it was shown that tinnitus prevalence was a positive function of age and reported noise exposure. Furthermore, age and noise exposure seemed to be independent additive determinants for the risk of having tinnitus in the population. Since then, those data have been extended by similar analyses of Phases I and II (Coles 1984b). They are shown here in Table 3.2. In all three phases there was a significant increase with age in the prevalence of tinnitus. This association was independent of the reported occupational noise history. The increased risk of tinnitus with a positive history of occupational noise exposure was approximately 1.7 across phase and age, and for the under-40 age group there was a consistently higher risk still, by a factor of about two.

Interpretation is complicated by the fact that the older a person becomes the more years he has had in which to have increased his total noise immission. Also, in the last two decades there has been increased use of ear protectors by noise-exposed workers; this will have substantially reduced the noise immissions, especially in the younger age groups. The trend is shown in Figure 3.1 in which Davis (1983a) has plotted the

Table 3.2 TINNITUS, AGE AND NOISE. Percentages of people reporting experience of tinnitus in each of 18 groups defined by age, history of occupational noise exposure and NSH phase. (Tinnitus of spontaneous type and of over 5 min duration. Combined Tier A data from the four cities. After Coles, 1984b).

Phase of NSH	Occupational noise exposure history	Age group (years)		
		<40	40–60	>60
Pilot	No	11.1	13.2	18.2
	Yes	21.9	21.4	32.8
I	No	5.8	10.1	14.4
	Yes	12.1	13.6	20.8
II	No	5.4	9.8	14.2
	Yes	11.0	17.1	23.5

percentage of people that fell into three categories of noise exposure (identified in detail at Tier B, with allowance for use of any ear protection) as a function of age. In the case of occupational noise exposure, there is a fairly steady increase in the percentage of noise-exposed people; 31% of the men were so exposed and 10% of the women. With respect to shooting and explosive noise exposure, 38.6% of the men and 1.5% of the women were so exposed. Peaks in the graph appear in the age groups 60–69 years and 80–89 years, which include the major groups affected by World Wars II and I respectively. On the other hand, social noise exposure is largely restricted to the younger groups, and was probably due mainly to amplified music.

There is much confounding of noise exposure with age and gender, and also with socio-economic group, the skilled manual and semi-skilled groups (socio-economic

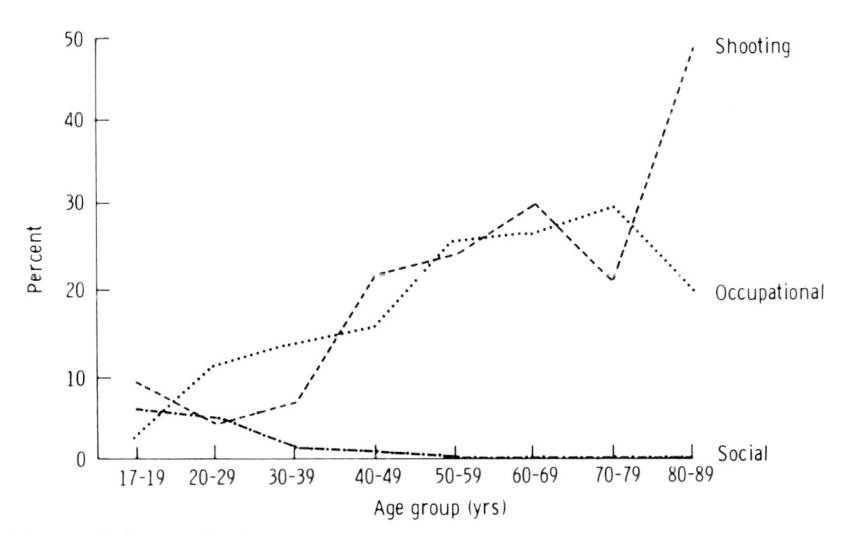

Fig. 3.1 Influences of noise, exposure and age. Percentage of people with significant unprotected shooting and explosive, occupational and social noise exposures in 8 age groups. (NSH Phases I and II, Tier B data from the 4 cities combined. After Davis, 1983a).

groups IIIM and IV in Fig. 3.3 below being those most likely to suffer industrial noise exposure. Unfortunately the population, and also the samples in Phases I and II, contains rather too few people with material noise exposure in certain age bands and socio-economic groups (e.g. young, non-manually employed females) to enable the effects of these tied variables to be untied. Nevertheless, the importance of noise exposure as one determinant of tinnitus enhances the case for further effort in health education and occupational health practice to reduce noise exposure. This modified case has been stated recently by Coles (1982) and Miller and Jakimetz (1984).

Gender

The percentages in each gender who reported tinnitus of spontaneous type and of duration over 5 minutes are shown in Table 3.3 for three NSH phases: Pilot, I and II. There was a small but significant trend for a higher prevalence of such tinnitus among females than among males. This has been reported in other population studies, e.g. those reviewed by Leske (1981) in the USA where 30% of males reported tinnitus (of any type) as compared with 35% of females, and in the OPCS study (1983) in the UK where 13% of males and 16% of females reported 'bothersome' tinnitus.

Table 3.3 TINNITUS AND GENDER. Percentages of people reporting tinnitus as a function of gender and NSH phase. (Tinnitus of spontaneous type and of over 5 min duration. Combined Tier A data from the four cities. After Coles, 1984b).

Phase	Male	Female
Pilot	16.9	17.7
I	10.3	11.5
II	10.2	11.0

The prevalence of spontaneous tinnitus of over 5 minutes' duration in Phases I and II is shown in Figure 3.2 separately for males and females in seven age groups. A greater prevalence of tinnitus among females than males in the lower age groups contrasts with a predominance among men at the higher age groups. This could be due to a greater tendency to report tinnitus in women, but counteracted increasingly with age by the greater noise exposure of men. The general increase of tinnitus with age is also illustrated.

In Phase I of the NSH, Davis (1983b) showed that a much higher proportion of females than males reported tinnitus that was severely annoying or that interfered with getting to sleep. The same trend is shown in Figure 3.3. A similar conclusion could also be drawn from the data reviewed by Leske (1981) where there was a greater relative difference between females and males reporting severe tinnitus than mild tinnitus.

It is interesting to speculate on the nature and causes of these gender differences. The prevalence of tinnitus, especially in its more severe degrees, could conceivably be higher in females than males; however, this cannot be taken as a serious working hypothesis in the absence of any reasonable explanatory mechanism. Studies collated by Robinson & Sutton (1979) on hearing threshold levels as a function of age and gender show that in all age groups females have rather better hearing above 1000 Hz

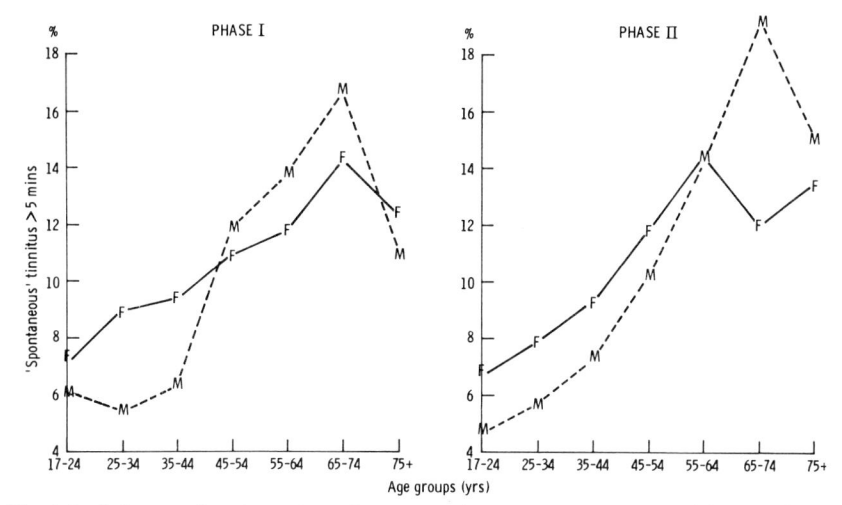

Fig. 3.2 Influence of gender and age. Prevalence of tinnitus in 7 age bands, with males (M) and females (F) shown separately. (Tinnitus of spontaneous type and of over 5 min duration. NSH Phases I and II, Tier A data from the 4 cities combined. After Coles, 1984b).

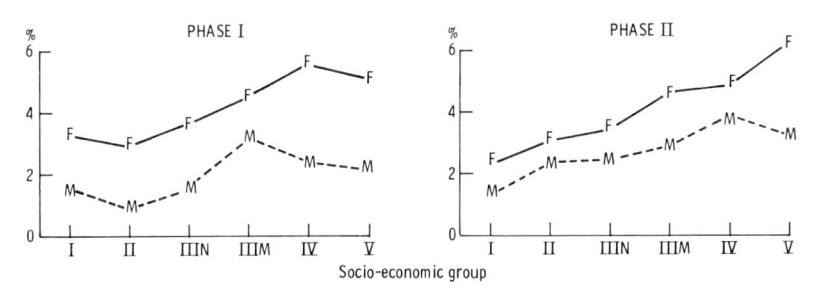

Fig. 3.3 Influence of socio-economic status and gender. Prevalence of tinnitus causing interference with getting to sleep in 6 socio-economic groups, with males (M) and females (F) shown separately. (Tinnitus of spontaneous type and over 5 min duration. NSH Phases I and II, Tier A data from the 4 cities combined. After Coles, 1984b).

than males. Greater noise exposure may account for much of the difference, to judge from two of the studies they quote (Hinchcliffe 1959, Hinchcliffe & Jones 1968). On the other hand, in the NSH females were found to have slightly better hearing above 500 Hz than males even when differences in age, socio-economic group and noise immission history were controlled for (Davis 1982). Thus, females' hearing is at least no worse than that of males. Since tinnitus is associated with hearing disorder and the severity of tinnitus is related to the degree of hearing loss (Coles & Davis 1983, Hazell et al 1985), it seems unlikely that females have any higher prevalence or severity of tinnitus. An alternative and more likely proposition is that females have a generally greater awareness of somatic symptoms, and for a given degree of unpleasant sensation tend to place it higher on scales describing severity and effects on well-being. Another possibility is that females' daily experience of distracting sounds or activities may be less. There is no way of determining the relative contributions of all these possibilities from the data currently available.

Socio-economic status (SES)

Figure 3.3 shows SES effects in those whose tinnitus caused interference with getting to sleep. Tinnitus reports rise from the professionally employed (I) to the unskilled occupations (V), with a fair degree of consistency between phases of the NSH. In groups IIIM and IV, where noise exposure is maximum, the male data do not climb to meet the female data; this suggests that SES conveys information about tinnitus additional to that of noise exposure.

GEOGRAPHICAL INFLUENCES

There were no consistent differences between phases in the overall prevalence of spontaneous tinnitus of over 5 minutes duration between the four cities sampled: Cardiff, Glasgow, Nottingham and Southampton. Also there were no differences between the prevalences in the four cities of tinnitus causing a severe effect on ability to lead a normal life or on quality of life.

CLINICAL FEATURES

Clinic populations

Presumably tinnitus clinic samples are drawn mainly from those with the more severe degrees of tinnitus. Discounting other influences, one might therefore expect from the data shown in Figure 3 that clinics would show a female-to-male ratio of about 3:2. Considering the greater longevity of females together with the increasing prevalence of tinnitus with age, an even higher ratio might be expected. Table 3.4 shows that this is not what actually happens. Over the period 1976–1981 in the largest tinnitus clinic in the USA, 68% of the patients were male, with females outnumbering males only in the over-70 age group (Meikle 1985). In a study of therapeutic masking based on three of the largest tinnitus clinics in UK, of the 472 new patients entered into the study (mostly in 1981-1982) 47% were male, with no apparent interaction between gender and age at first attendance (Hazell et al 1985).

Table 3.4 AGE AT FIRST TINNITUS CLINIC ATTENDANCE. (After Meikle 1985, and Hazell et al 1985).

	Meikle (1985) ($n=1725$)		Hazell et al (1985) ($n=472$)		
Age band (years)	% of sample	Male:female (%) ($n=1182:543$)	Age band (years)	% of sample	Male:female (%) ($n=223:249$)
<21	3	66:34	<20	2	50:50
21-30	6	72:28	20-29	2	55:45
31-40	13	80:20	30-39	9	45:55
41-50	17	76:24	40-49	14	50:50
51-60	28	71:29	50-59	32	47:53
61-70	23	63:37	60-69	32	44:56
>70	10	45:55	>69	9	56:46
All	100	68:32	All	100	47:53

Two factors may have biased the British sample towards a relatively larger proportion of female and/or elderly patients. One was the inclusion of a number of self-referrals by members of the local branch of the British Tinnitus Association in the Nottingham sub-sample and a less direct influence of the Association in a significant proportion of the referrals to all three centres. This notion is supported by recent changes in the patient clientèle at the Nottingham tinnitus clinic. 128 new patients were entered from Nottingham into the Hazell et al (1985) study, in the period January 1981 to March 1983. Since then, 133 new patients were seen in the period April 1983 to April 1984, and another 152 from May 1984 to April 1985. In the DHSS study, the age at attendance was maximal in the 60–70 years age group and 44% were male: in the 1983 to 1984 clinics, the age at attendance was maximal equally in the 50–59 and 60-69 years age groups and 46% were male: in the 1984 to 1985 clinics, the age of attendance was maximal in the 50–59 years age group and 51% were male.

The other potential bias lay in the possible exclusion from the study, which involved a commitment to multiple attendances, of more males than females. Of 668 new patients at the three centres, 196 were excluded from the study. The reasons are listed in Hazell et al's (1985) Table 4, but unfortunately information on their distribution as a function of gender is not available.

There seem to be two possible explanations for this underlying predominance of male referrals. The first is economic. Because tinnitus interferes with thought processes and getting to sleep and causes irritability and tension, it may threaten occupational efficiency and job security. This will often be a more serious matter for men, and especially in young and early middle ages. The other possible explanation is somewhat akin (but in the opposite direction) to that offered to explain the apparently higher prevalence of tinnitus in females. That is, whilst females may have a greater awareness of somatic symptoms and describe them in terms of greater severity, males may have a lower threshold of discomfort at which they will seek professional advice. It is not possible to say whether either of these two explanations is correct; quite possibly both are to some extent.

Other factors of interest in comparing population prevalence and clinic attendance rates are socio-economic status (SES) and age. With respect to SES, a direct comparison is made in the Hazell et al report (1985) (Table 3.5) in which there is a small but consistent tendency for a disproportionately higher attendance rate from the

Table 3.5 INTERVAL BETWEEN ONSET AND TINNITUS CLINIC ATTENDANCE. Percentages by age band. (After Meikle 1985, and Hazell et al 1985)

	Meikle (1985) n=1561, seen 1976–1981					Hazell et al (1985)			
		n=288, seen ca. 1984				n=465, seen 1981–1983			
		Age (years) at first attendance:							
Interval (years)	All	<41 (n=67)	41–60 (n=126)	>60 (n=95)	All	<41 (n=59)	41–60 (n=234)	>60 (n=172)	All
<1	15	22	19	22	21	22	13	10	15
1–5	38	34	32	21	29	47	51	36	45
>5	47	43	49	57	50	31	32	53	40

better paid occupations. This is in keeping with the influence of the socio-economic factors on uptake of health services generally, as discussed recently in the audiological context by Haggard & Armstrong-Bednall (1984).

The ages at which patients first attended tinnitus clinics in the USA and UK (Table 3.4) may be compared with statistics on tinnitus in the population as a whole, derived from the NSH. Of particular interest is the age distribution in the general population of those who had consulted their general practitioner (GP) or attended a hospital clinic about their tinnitus (Coles & Davis 1983, Fig. 10). Of those reporting severely annoying tinnitus the percentage who had consulted their GP about it rose fairly steadily with age, perhaps reflecting a constant incidence rate for tinnitus of this degree leading to a cumulatively rising prevalence with age. In contrast, the percentage who had attended a hospital clinic about their tinnitus rose sharply after the age of 40, perhaps indicating the forties as an age when tinnitus is most worrying. This supposition is borne out in Figure 7 of the paper by Coles & Davis (1983), in which the percentages of people (at tier A in Phases I, II and III) who reported tinnitus as having a severe effect on the quality of their life rose sharply after the age of 40 years in the females and 50 in the males.

The question then arises as to the age at which the incidence of tinnitus is maximal. It could be inferred retrospectively from much of the NSH data on prevalence of tinnitus in the general population that there is either a gradually increasing incidence with age or a tendency to an increased incidence after 40 years of age. Some further information comes from the tinnitus sub-study of Phase III where, in the 62 persons in the Nottingham sample seen at Tier B, the distribution of ages on onset peaked markedly in the 51–60 years age group for males but suggested a more widespread range of maximum incidence (covering three decades after 40 years of age) in females.

Data are also available for the incidence of tinnitus in particular populations. Merluzzi et al (1983) have reported on 577 males working in tramcar body repair shops, of whom 34% had noise-induced hearing loss and 25% other causes of hearing loss. 28% of the men reported tinnitus, with the distribution of ages of onset maximal in the 40–44 years age group.

In the American and British tinnitus clinic samples information on age of onset was not available directly, but can be estimated somewhat approximately from the data on age of first attendance (Table 3.4) and interval between onset and first attendance (Table 3.5). The American data show greatest attendance in the 51–60 years age group with the most common interval being over 5 years, which suggests an onset of tinnitus maximal in the later forties. The British data show greatest attendance in the 50–59 and 60–69 years age groups, with a most common interval of 1–5 years, which suggests an onset of tinnitus maximal in the later fifties.

Table 3.5 also shows that there is no important interaction between the age of onset of tinnitus and the onset/first-attendance interval. Therefore we must look to other factors to explain the differences in the pattern of referral to the American and British tinnitus clinics. The fact that the American attenders have such a predominance of males, in all but the over-70 age group, may reflect greater economic pressures and lesser occupational security in that country. Likewise the potentially greater economic threat posed by tinnitus to American patients could account for the slightly younger age of first attendance there. At first sight the longer interval between onset of tinnitus and attendance at the American tinnitus clinic might seem to contradict this explanation, but that effect is probably explained by the vast distances that many of the patients have to travel (from all over the country and from other American countries to the particular clinic in the North-Western corner of the USA). It is possibly influenced also by the financial disincentive for referral of patients from one ENT specialist to another in the USA.

It is appropriate also to look at changes in referral pattern. With respect to the Portland tinnitus clinic, Meikle (1985) has noted that 'the recent surge of clinical interest in tinnitus, which dates from about 1976 in this country [i.e. the USA], has caused many people to come in to the clinics who previously did not know there were such services available. We believe we have been dealing with a large "backlog" of patients who have had tinnitus for years, and that . . . the figures will change in regard to duration of tinnitus prior to the first clinic visit. In fact, already we believe we are seeing . . . proportionately more of the recent onset cases'. That impression would seem to be supported by the more recent data provided by her, which are included in Table 3.5. Moreover, in the UK, a similar change towards more recent-onset cases has been noted recently (Coles 1985) in the patients referred to the Nottingham tinnitus clinic which was one of the three in the Hazell et al (1985) study.

Broadly speaking, the statistics on tinnitus in the general population and in the clinic samples are compatible one with the other. The study of the common and the discrepant trends yields information important both for the planning of services for tinnitus and as a background to conclusions concerning aetiology and treatment that may be drawn from research on different types of sample.

Site of tinnitus

Clinical reports have indicated that tinnitus affects the left ear rather more commonly than the right, e.g. Hazell et al (1981, 1985), Meikle & Taylor-Walsh (1984). But only a marginally greater prevalence of tinnitus on the left side, and in males only, has been found in studies of the general population; see Table 3.6 below for data from Phases I and II of the NSH. The Pilot Study had already given somewhat similar overall percentages which suggested further analyses, some of which have already been reported (Institute of Hearing Research 1981b). One interesting idea was that the difference was mediated by handedness. 93% described themselves as right handed (defined by their reported use of their right hand for writing) and 7% as left-handed.

Table 3.6 SITE OF TINNITUS. Percentages of males and females reporting particular sites of tinnitus. (Tinnitus of spontaneous type and of over 5 min duration. NSH Tier A data from Phase I and II combined, from the four cities combined. After Coles, 1984b).

	Tinnitus site		
	Mostly left	Mostly right	Both ears or in the head
Females (n=882)	25	26	49
Males (n=696)	29	24	47

Tinnitus was reported by 17.9% of the right-handed and 14.8% of the left-handed, a significant difference. But, as expected (Fleminger et al 1977), this report of handedness was age-dependent: use of left hand for writing was reported by approximately 10, 6 and 3% in the age groups of under-40, 40–60 and over 60 years respectively in each of the NSH phases discussed here. Once age effects were controlled, handedness was shown not to be a significant factor in explaining tinnitus laterality ($p > 0.1$, Phases I and II).

Another possible explanation for more frequent tinnitus on the left side was asymmetric noise exposure, notably from shooting with a rifle or shotgun, which is usually from the right shoulder. However, analyses of Tier B data in Phase II showed no correlation between side of tinnitus and side of asymmetric noise exposure, either military or industrial, a finding in keeping with that of Hallam et al (1984).

Pitch and loudness: scaling and matching

Tinnitus measurements in the NSH have been somewhat limited prior to the present Phase III. In spite of this, some useful findings emerged from the measurements performed in Phase II. Subjects with tinnitus were asked to rate the pitch and loudness of their tinnitus on a scale from 1 to 10, and to match its pitch and loudness with pure tones generated by an audiometer. As might be expected the pitch scaling correlated significantly with the pitch matching, although not to a useful degree ($r=0.31$, $p>0.001$). Loudness rating correlated significantly with the loudness matching, when the latter was expressed in decibels HL (hearing level) ($r=0.37$; $p<0.001$). Interestingly however, when the loudness matches were expressed in sensation level (SL) re threshold at the tinnitus frequency, the correlation coefficient was negligible ($r = 0.03$). Such a discrepancy has been reported several times previously (Evered & Lawrenson 1981; Hazell 1981; Tyler & Conrad-Armes 1983; Hazell et al 1985), and is a further instance of the generally scant value of scales based on SL for describing loudness in sensorineural conditions, and should discourage any further description of *loudness* of tinnitus being expressed in dB SL.

Unexpectedly, the highest correlation was between the loudness scaling and the pitch scaling ($r=0.51, p<0.001$). Some correlation between pitch and loudness might be expected: hearing losses of tinnitus patients are generally greater at higher frequencies, and tinnitus generally is more severe the greater the hearing loss (Hazell et al 1985). However, the correlation coefficient of 0.31 between the loudness scaling and the loudness matching (expressed in dB HL) suggests that there is a second factor accounting for the correlation coefficient of 0.51 between the pitch and loudness scalings. It seems that many people do not use the word 'pitch' in its precise musical or psychophysical sense and tend to use it as an indicator of how high on the *loudness* scale the sound is 'pitched', i.e. located. This could also explain the surprisingly low correlation noted above between pitch scaling and pitch matching. In fact timbre (which is only equivalent to pitch in the special case of pure tones) is a more appropriate descriptive term for this aspect of tinnitus quality: but unfortunately timbre is a word even less understood by the general public. Clearly, when taking a history and seeking to ascertain the frequency zone of a tinnitus sound, the clinician should use the words which best elicit in the dialect of the patient the concept of timbre, such as 'sharp' or 'whistling' versus 'dull' or 'roaring'.

Pathological correlates

In the NSH an attempt was made to tie down casual factors or correlated disease states by taking comprehensive clinical histories and a considerable number of measures of general health. Analyses with respect to hearing measurements and tinnitus have so far been limited to the hearing threshold level (HTL) data, but these are of likely relevance to tinnitus also. Coles (1984b) reported that only somewhat borderline correlations with HTL, mostly with no aetiologically inviting interpretation, were found for: 1. history of cardiovascular disorder; 2. systolic and diastolic blood pressure; and 3. current use of beta-blocker drugs and loop diuretics. Of course the former group of drugs, and to some extent the latter too, are taken because of cardiovascular disorders, which could themselves have contributed to the causation of the hearing disorder. Non-significant correlations were obtained between HTL and present or past alcohol consumption and a variety of other drugs which many of the subjects were currently taking.

A range of haematological tests, liver, thyroid and renal function tests, general blood chemistry and serological tests for syphilis were also carried out, but no correlation repeatable between phases was found between tinnitus and the results of these tests. Similar null results were found for associations with hearing impairment. On the other hand, Browning et al (1986) report that further analyses of NSH data using the ratio between total protein and the albumin fraction, which provides an indirect measure of plasma viscosity, support their other study with ENT clinic patients suggesting a substantial correlation between the rheological properties of blood and the degree of sensorineural hearing loss.

An example of the clinical relevance of these otherwise null results is given by the syphilis serology tests. These were only positive in 9 out of 1171 persons so tested. Of the 9, 7 had hearing within the range expected from their age, gender, noise exposure, and socio-economic status: the remaining 2 had middle ear pathology. The clinician faced with a patient with sensorineural hearing loss of unknown aetiology, on finding a positive syphilis serology, would tend in most circumstances to attribute the hearing disorder to syphilis. On the present evidence such action would not seem to be justified.

The lack of association of either tinnitus or HTL with the results of the various blood tests suggests that the conditions to which those tests are sensitive are not important determinants of tinnitus and/or hearing impairment in the population at large. Nevertheless, such blood tests, together with general clinical history and examination, continue to be useful investigations of particular patients with hearing disorders. A large literature suggests associations of hearing disorders with a wide variety of haematological disorders, hormonal disorders such as diabetes and hypothyroidism, bone disorders such as Paget's disease, and syphilis. Even if carefully controlled studies were eventually to show that these associations were marginal, the tests would still serve two other functions. They may indicate possible predisposing, synergistic or precipitating factors interacting with other known or unknown causes of hearing disorder. They may also identify conditions needing treatment in their own right. This in turn may lessen the handicapping or distressing effect of the coincident hearing disorder or tinnitus.

Natural history of tinnitus

Every tinnitus patient wants to know whether his tinnitus will get better or worse. Up to now research has not provided any guidance and consequently the information given to the patient has tended to reflect the clinician's personal experience of patients, particularly those seen by him on two or more occasions. These will tend to be the people who have adapted less well to a continuous tinnitus and demand further attention, in turn leading possibly to a pessimistic bias concerning prognosis.

Some interim information on a population sample of the type required for more informed counselling is now available from Phase III of the NSH. Tier A questionnaires (see Appendix 3.1) were sent to 25 642 people; replies were received from 18 677, with 17 238 remaining after exclusion of those with missing data. Of these, 8045 (46.7%) replied (Yes) to the question 'Have you ever had noises in your head or ears?', and 6063 (35.2%) went on to answer yes to the question 'Nowadays do you get noises in your head or ears?'. The important feature with respect to tinnitus natural history is that of the 8045 who had at one time experienced tinnitus, 1982 (24.6%) did not get it 'nowadays'. However, before more explicit counselling can be given we need a breakdown of this figure in terms of duration, intermittency and various grades of severity of the former tinnitus. This is being obtained in Phase III (Tier B of which was not complete at the time of writing).

The other information needed clinically concerns the time course of loudness and severity of tinnitus that persists. Some limited data are available from the 61 people in the Nottingham sample of the tinnitus sub-study. These were selected in the first place from responses at Tier A (see Appendix 3.1, Phase III) to question B2 indicating that tinnitus was present nowadays for most of the time, to question B7 indicating tinnitus was present at least half of the time, and to question B6 indicating that the tinnitus was slightly, moderately or severely annoying. The group comprised 37 males (mean age 59 years, limits 21–79) and 24 females (mean age 63 years, limits 22–79). The mean duration of the tinnitus they reported was 7 years, with none less than 2 years.

The relevant parts of the clinical data sheet (CDS) used at Tier B are given in Appendix 3.2. The results of CDS sections 2.6 (time course of loudness), 2.7 (time course of annoyance) and 2.8 (time course of sleep interference) have been analysed in order to meet the needs of this chapter. Table 3.7 shows the overall statistics on these three aspects of tinnitus natural history. Figures 3.4, 3.5 and 3.6 illustrate them graphically and give more information on the individual changes between different stages of the overall time course, arbitrarily defined as onset, middle and recently.

From these general population data, it would appear that tinnitus comes on suddenly subsequently alters little in loudness, although a proportion (28% in this sample) of those that come on gradually tend to go on increasing in loudness. On the

Table 3.7 NATURAL HISTORY OF TINNITUS. Overall statistics. (NSH Phase III, Tier B data from Nottingham sample of tinnitus sub-study).

	Period in tinnitus history		
	Onset	Middle	Recently
Loudness changes (valid data on 59 subjects)			
Increasing	[1]	14 (24%)	13 (22%)
Unchanging		43 (73%)	42 (71%)
Decreasing		2 (3%)	3 (5%)
Ended		0	1 (2%)
Annoyance (valid data on 61 subjects)			
None	20 (33%)	26 (43%)	27 (44%)
Slight	24 (39%)	22 (36%)	21 (34%)
Moderate	12 (20%)	11 (18%)	8 (13%)
Severe	5 (8%)	2 (3%)	5 (8%)
Sleep disturbance (valid data on 59 subjects)			
No	45 (76%)	47 (80%)	45 (76%)
Yes	14 (24%)	12 (20%)	14 (24%)

[1] Sudden onset 23, gradual onset 36

other hand, there may be a slight tendency (not reaching statistical significance with these limited data) towards reduction of annoyance after the onset period, although there is little change after that. This fits clinical experience of many patients learning to live with their tinnitus after an initial period of discomfort and anxiety. Indeed, some tinnitus clinic patients actually report increasing loudness but decreasing annoyance, and a somewhat similar trend is seen in the population statistics (compare Figs. 3.4c and 3.5c). In contrast, the proportion of persons experiencing sleep disturbance appears to remain much the same throughout.

Until we have more detailed information it would thus seem reasonable to counsel people with tinnitus, regarding prognosis, as follows: 'The general pattern of severity is likely to stay much as it is now, or slightly decrease. It is unlikely to get markedly worse, although that does occasionally happen: sometimes it gets markedly better, or may even disappear altogether'.

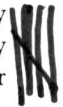

Many tinnitus sufferers do not like being told baldly that they have got to learn to live with their tinnitus, and attention has to be given to the way the message is expressed. But there does seem to be a tendency towards habituation. Likewise, it would not be reassuring to tell those with gradual onset of tinnitus that some of them will experience a further growth of loudness. To a considerable degree it appears that the latter process, perhaps representing the effects of progressive pathology, is more than counteracted by the tendency towards habituation. Hence the prognosis above has been expressed in the more collective term of 'severity' when it can truthfully be the guardedly reassuring one given above.

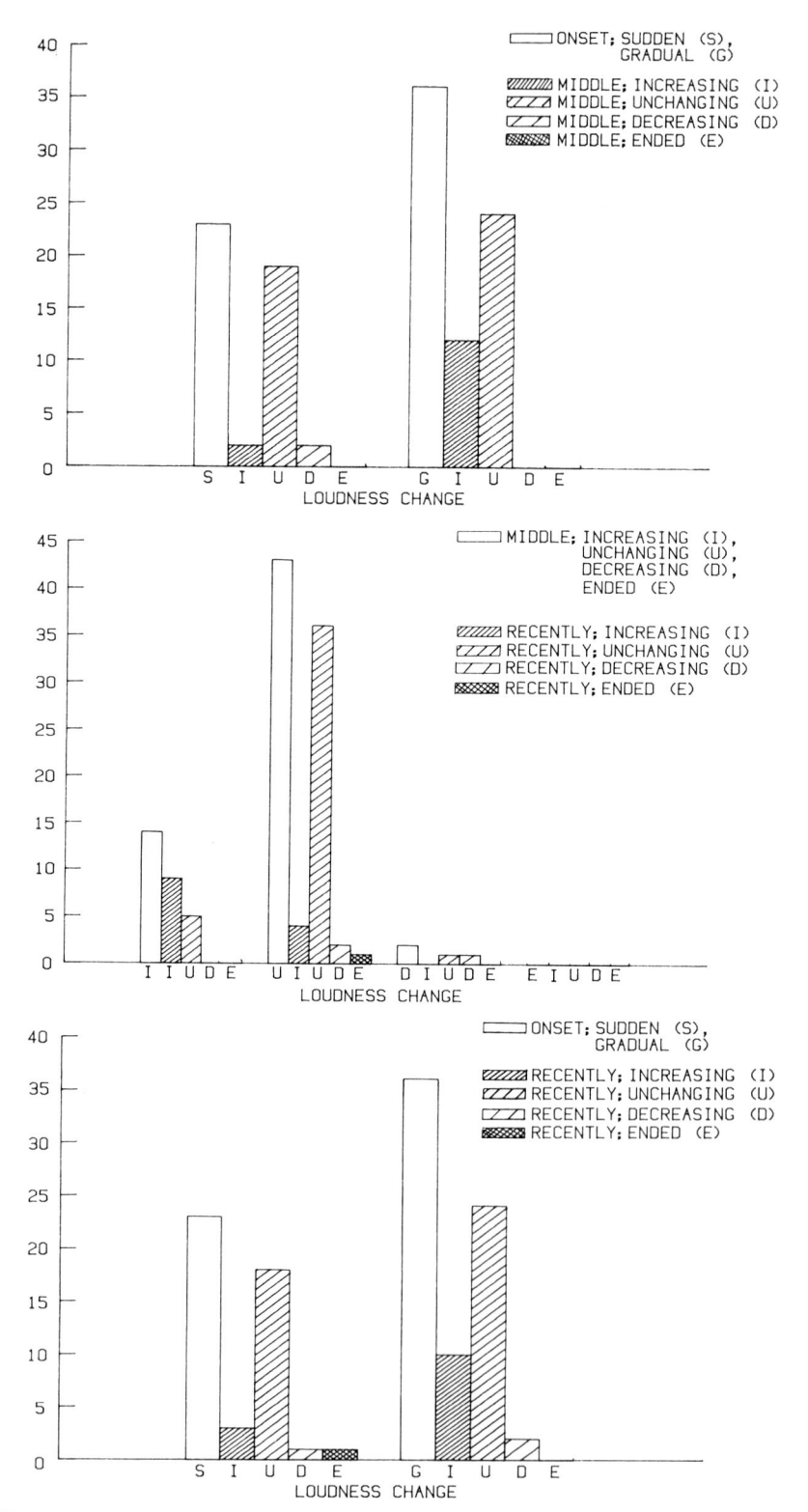

Fig. 3.4 Time course of loudness of tinnitus. a. Onset to middle b. middle to recently c. onset to recently. Ordinates: numbers of subjects. (NSH Phase III, Tier B data from the Nottingham sample of tinnitus sub-study).

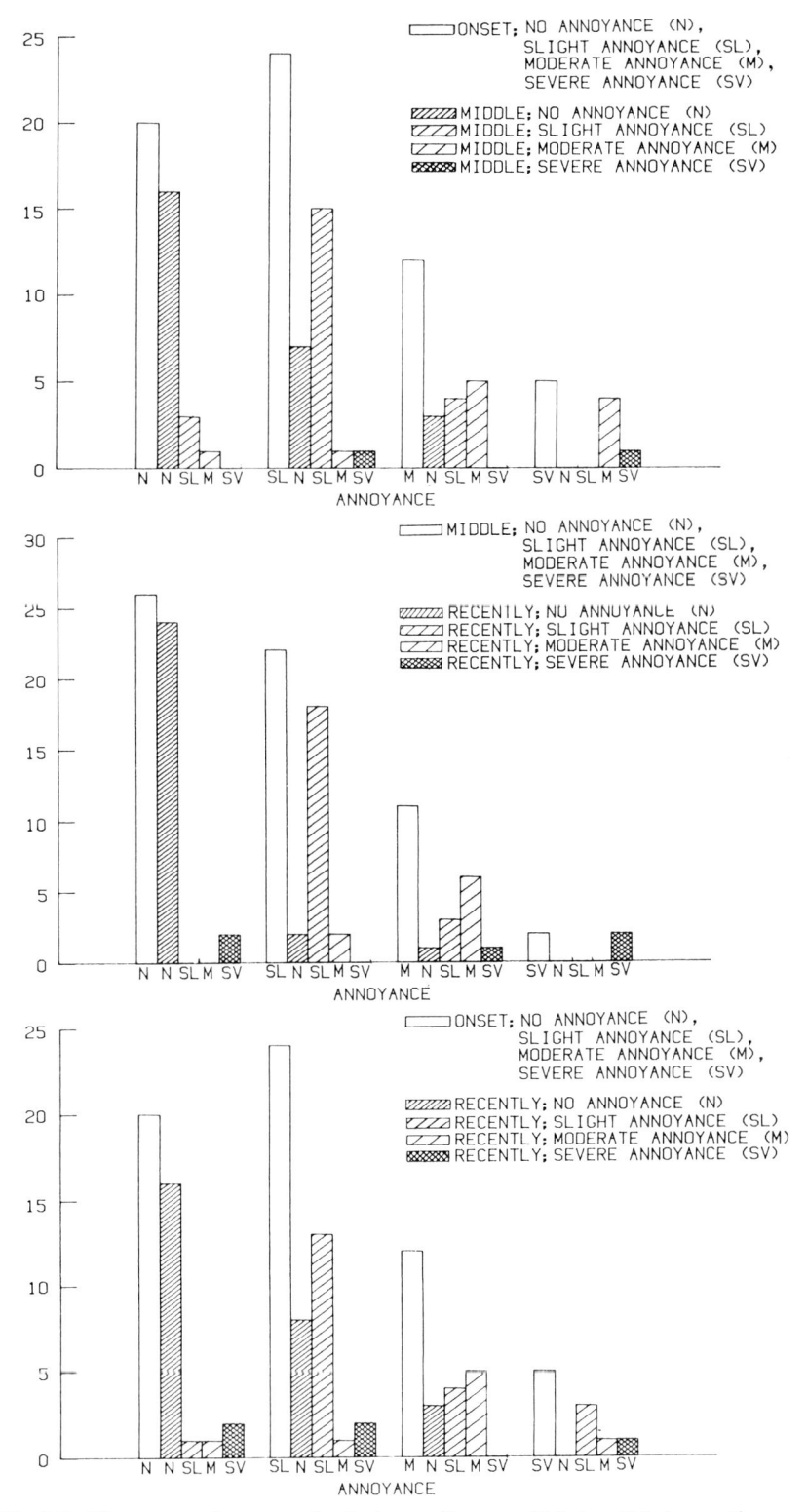

Fig. 3.5 Time course of annoyance by tinnitus. a. Onset to middle b. middle to recently c. onset to recently. Ordinates: numbers of subjects. (NSH Phase III, Tier B data from the Nottingham sample of tinnitus sub-study).

Sleep Disturbance	Onset	Middle	Recently
No	45 ———→ 41 ——(36)——→ 38		
	(5) ╳		
	(2) ╱		
Yes	(see below)	4 ——(2)——→ 7	

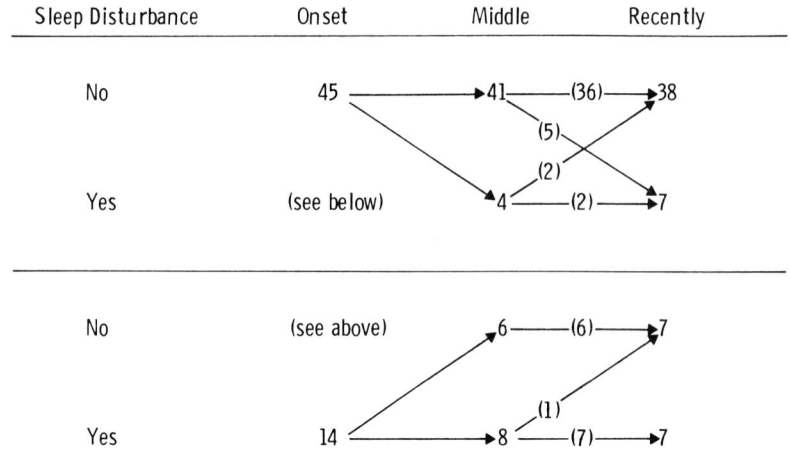

No	(see above)	6 ——(6)——→ 7	
	(1) ╱		
Yes	14 ———→ 8 ——(7)——→ 7		

Fig. 3.6 Time course of sleep disturbance by tinnitus. Numerals represent numbers of subjects. (NSH Phase III, Tier B data from the Nottingham sample of tinnitus sub-study).

REFERENCES

Browning G G, Gatehouse S, Lowe G D O 1986 Blood viscosity as a factor in sensorineural hearing impairment. Lancet i: 121–123

Coles R R A 1982 Noise-induced tinnitus. Proceedings of the Institute of Acoustics, Bournemouth, 1982 (Liverpool): Institute of Acoustics pp G4.1–G4.5

Coles R R A 1984a Epidemiology of tinnitus: (1) prevalence. Journal of Laryngology and Otology Supplement 9: 7–15

Coles R R A 1948b Epidemiology of tinnitus: (2) demographic and clinical features. Journal of Laryngology and Otology Supplement 9: 195–202

Coles R R A 1985 Personal communication

Coles R R A, Davis A C 1983 Tinnitus and ageing. Unpublished paper to the British Society of Audiology (text available from the second author at the Institute of Hearing Research). Quoted by Coles et al (1985).

Coles R R A, Baskill J L, Sheldrake J B 1985 Measurement and management of tinnitus. II, Management. Journal of Laryngology and Otology 99: 1–10 [see Fig. 1]

Davis A C 1982 The National Study of Hearing. Prevalence and population parameters of auditory impairment in the adult population of Great Britain. Unpublished paper to the Epidemiology Section of the Royal Society of Medicine (text available from the author at the Insitute of Hearing Research)

Davis A C 1983a Effects of noise and socioeconomic factors on hearing impairment. In: Rossi G (ed) Noise as a public health problem, Vol 1: Proceedings of 4th International Congress. Edizioni Techniche a cura del Centro Ricerche e Studi Amplifon, Milan, pp 201–211

Davis A C 1983b Hearing disorders in the population: first phase findings of the MRC National Study of Hearing. In: Lutman M E, Haggard M P (eds) Hearing science and hearing disorders. Academic Press, London, pp 35–60

Evered D, Lawrenson G (eds) 1981 Guidelines for recommended procedures in tinnitus testing. In: Tinnitus: Ciba Foundation Symposium 85. Pitman, London. Appendix III, pp 303–306

Fleminger J J, Dalton R, Standage K J 1977 Age as a factor in the handedness of adults. Neuropsychologia 15: 471–473

Haggard M P, Armstrong-Bednall G 1984 Requirements of structure and resource for an adequate audiology service in the post-Griffiths Health Service. British Journal of Audiology 18: 183-194

Hallam R S, Rachman S, Hinchcliffe R 1984 Psychological aspects of tinnitus. In: Rachman S (ed) Contributions to medical psychology, Vol 3. Pergamon, Oxford, pp 31–54

Hazell J W P 1981 Measurement of tinnitus in humans. In: Evered D, Lawrenson G (eds) Tinnitus: Ciba Foundation Symposium 85. Pitman, London, pp 35–53

Hazell J W P, Williams G R, Sheldrake J B 1981 Tinnitus maskers–successes and failures: a report on the state of the art. Journal of Laryngology and Otology Supplement 4: 80–87

Hazell J W P, Wood S M, Cooper H R et al 1985 A clinical study of tinnitus maskers. British Journal of Audiology 19: 64–146

Hinchcliffe R 1959 The threshold of hearing as a function of age. Acustica 9: 303–308

Hinchcliffe R 1961 Prevalence of the commoner ear, nose and throat conditions in the adult rural population of Great Britain. British Journal of Preventive and Social Medicine 15: 128–140

Hinchcliffe R, Jones W I 1968 Hearing levels of a suburban Jamaican population. International Audiology 7: 239–258

Institute of Hearing Research 1981a Population study of hearing disorders in adults: preliminary communication. Journal of the Royal Society of Medicine 74: 819–827

Institute of Hearing Research 1981b Epidemiology of tinnitus. In: Evered D, Lawrenson G (eds) Tinnitus: Ciba Foundation Symposium 85. Pitman, London, pp 16–34

Leske M C 1981 Prevalence estimates of communicative disorder in the US: language, hearing and vestibular disorders. Asha 23: 229–237

Meikle M 1985 Personal communication

Meikle M, Taylor-Walsh E 1984 Characteristics of tinnitus and related observations in over 1800 tinnitus clinic patients. Journal of Laryngology and Otology Supplement 9: 17–21

Merluzzi F, Duca P G, Ciuffreda M, di Credico N, Cantoni S 1983. Tinnitus and occupational exposure to noise. In: Rossi G (ed) Noise as a public health problem, Vol 1: Proceedings of 4th International Congress, Edizioni Techniche a cura del Centro Ricerche e Studi Amplifon, Milan, pp 377–380

Miller M H, Jakimetz J R 1984 Noise exposure, hearing loss, speech discrimination and tinnitus. Journal of Laryngology and Otology Supplement 9: 74–76

Office of Population Censuses and Surveys 1983 General Household Survey. The prevalence of tinnitus 1981. OPCS Monitor. GHS 83/1, OPCS, London

Robinson D W, Sutton G J 1979 Age effect in hearing–a comparative analysis of published threshold data. Audiology 18: 320–334

Tyler R S, Conrad-Armes D 1983 The determination of tinnitus loudness considering the effects of recruitment. Journal of Speech and Hearing Research 26: 59–72

APPENDIX 3.1

National Study of Hearing, Pilot Phase and Phases I, II and III

Tinnitus sections in Tier A postal questionnaire (answered by the subjects and returned)

PILOT PHASE

In this section we are interested in whether you get ringing or buzzing noises in your head or ears. The occasional whistling or ringing in the ears of less than 5 minutes duration should *not* be counted. Also do *not* count those times when this happens just after very loud sounds, e.g. discos, shooting, or noise at work.

If you DO NOT get noises in your head or ears turn to SECTION C.

B1. Where do you most commonly hear buzzing or ringing in your head or ears?
  a. IN THE LEFT EAR
  b. IN THE RIGHT EAR
  c. IN BOTH EARS
  d. IN THE HEAD

B2. Indicate how annoying you find noises in your head or ears.
  a. NOT ANNOYING AT ALL
  b. ANNOYING TO A SLIGHT DEGREE
  c. ANNOYING TO A MODERATE DEGREE
  d. ANNOYING TO A SEVERE DEGREE

B3. Indicate to what extent noises in your head or ears affect your ability to lead a normal life.
  a. NOT AT ALL
  b. TO A SLIGHT DEGREE
  c. TO A MODERATE DEGREE
  d. TO A SEVERE DEGREE

B4. Do you ever get a buzzing or ringing noise in your head or ears that interferes with your getting to sleep?
  YES   NO

PHASE I

In this section we are interested in whether you get noises in your head or ears such as ringing or buzzing.

B1. Do you ever get any noises in your head or ears?
  YES   NO

If you never get noises in your head or ears please go to Section C.

B2. Do these noises usually last for longer than 5 minutes?
  YES   NO

B3. Do you hear these noises only following very loud sounds (e.g. discos, shooting or noise at work)?
  a. AFTER LOUD SOUNDS ONLY
  b. AT OTHER TIMES ONLY
  c. BOTH AFTER LOUD SOUNDS AND AT OTHER TIMES

B4. In which ear are you most affected by these noises?
  a. MOSTLY IN THE LEFT EAR
  b. MOSTLY IN THE RIGHT EAR
  c. EQUALLY IN BOTH EARS OR IN THE HEAD

B5. Indicate how the noises in your head or ears change when you are in a noisy place.
   a. THEY BECOME MORE NOTICEABLE
   b. THEY STAY ABOUT THE SAME
   c. THEY BECOME LESS NOTICEABLE

B6. Indicate how *annoying* you find the noises in your head or ears.
   a. NOT ANNOYING AT ALL
   b. SLIGHTLY ANNOYING
   c. MODERATELY ANNOYING
   d. SEVERELY ANNOYING

B7. Do the noises in your head or ears ever interfere with your getting to sleep?
   YES   NO

PHASE II

In this section we are interested in whether you get noises in your head or ears such as ringing or buzzing.

B1. Nowadays do you ever get noises in your head or ears?
   a. YES, MOST OF THE TIME
   b. YES, SOME OF THE TIME
   c. NO

If you do not get noises in your head or ears please go to Section C.

B2. Do these noises usually last for longer than 5 minutes?
   YES   NO

B3. Do you hear these noises only following very loud sounds (e.g. discos, shooting or noise at work)?
   a. AFTER LOUD SOUNDS ONLY
   b. AT OTHER TIMES ONLY
   c. BOTH AFTER LOUD SOUNDS AND AT OTHER TIMES

B4. In which ear are you most affected by these noises?
   a. MOSTLY IN THE LEFT EAR
   b. MOSTLY IN THE RIGHT EAR
   c. EQUALLY IN BOTH EARS OR IN THE HEAD

B5. Indicate how the noises in your head or ears change when you are in a noisy place.
   a. THEY BECOME MORE NOTICEABLE
   b. THEY STAY ABOUT THE SAME
   c. THEY BECOME LESS NOTICEABLE.

B6. Indicate how *annoying* you find the noises in your head or ears when they are at their loudest.
   a. NOT ANNOYING AT ALL
   b. SLIGHTLY ANNOYING
   c. MODERATELY ANNOYING
   d. SEVERELY ANNOYING

B7. Indicate to what extent the noises in your head or ears affect the quality of your life as a whole.
   a. NOT AT ALL
   b. TO A SLIGHT DEGREE
   c. TO A MODERATE DEGREE
   d. TO A SEVERE DEGREE

B8. Do the noises in your head or ears ever interfere with your getting to sleep?
   YES   NO

PHASE III

Many people get noises in their head or ears such as ringing, buzzing or whistling. In this section we are interested in whether YOU do.

B1. Have you ever had noises in your head or ears?
  a. NO
  b. YES

B2. Nowadays do you get noises in your head or ears?
  a. NO
  b. YES, SOME OF THE TIME
  c. YES, MOST OF THE TIME

B3. Do these noises usually last for longer than 5 minutes?
  a. NO
  b. YES

B4. When do you get these noises?
  a. ONLY AFTER LOUD SOUNDS (e.g. shooting, discos, noise at work)
  b. ONLY AT OTHER TIMES
  c. BOTH AFTER LOUD SOUNDS AND AT OTHER TIMES

B5. In which ear or side of the head are you most affected by these noises?
  a. EQUALLY IN BOTH EARS OR IN THE MIDDLE OF THE HEAD
  b. MORE ON THE RIGHT
  c. MORE ON THE LEFT

B6. Indicate how ANNOYING you find the noises in your ears or head when they are at their worst.
  a. SEVERELY ANNOYING
  b. MODERATELY ANNOYING
  c. SLIGHTLY ANNOYING
  d. NOT AT ALL ANNOYING

B7. When you are awake and it is quiet, how much of the time are the noises in your head or ears present?
  a. A SMALL PART OF THE TIME
  b. ABOUT HALF THE TIME
  c. MOST OF THE TIME
  d. ALL THE TIME

APPENDIX 3.2

National Study of Hearing, Phase III. Tinnitus section of Tier B clinical data sheet
(recorded by the examining otologist or audiologist)

TINNITUS (spontaneous, over 5 min duration)

2.1 PRESENCE	Never (see definition of tinnitus)	0
	Nowadays, some of the time (see def.)	1
	Nowadays, most of the time (see def.)	2
	Previously, some of the time	3
	Prevoiuysly, most of the time	4
	Don't know	D
2.2 SIDE	Never had tinnitus	N
(of most troublesome noises present nowadays,	Right, or mostly right	1
or previously if not present)	Left, or mostly left	2
	Central, or equal R & L	3
	Don't know	D
2.3 OCCURRENCE OF BOUTS	Never had tinnitus	N
(see definition)	Not in bouts	1
(of most troublesome noises present nowadays,	Everyday or nearly	2
or previously if not present) 'How often do	3-4 times a week	3
you usually hear the noises nowadays?' or	Once or twice a week	4
if not present nowadays: 'How often did you	Once or twice a month	5
usually hear the noises when you had them	Very variable	6
previously?'	Other (specify ....)	8
	Don't know	D
2.4 DURATION OF BOUTS (see definition)	Never had tinnitus	N
(of most troublesome noises present nowadays,	Not in bouts	1
or previously if not present) 'How long do the	5 to 25 minutes	2
noises usually last nowadays?' or if not present	25 min–23 h	3
nowadays: 'How long did the noises usually	1, or more days	4
last when you had them previously?'	Very variable	5
	Other (specify ....)	8
	Don't know	D
2.5 LENGTH OF TINNITUS HISTORY	Never had tinnitus	N
(of any tinnitus) years ____	Enter number of years, rounded to the nearest year (1–5 months rounded down)	
	Don't know	D
2.6 OVERALL LOUDNESS HISTORY	Never had tinnitus	N
ONSET ____	Sudden onset	1
	Gradual onset or increase	2
MIDDLE ____	No general change	3
	Gradual decrease or end	4
RECENT OR END ____	Sudden end	5
	Don't know	D
2.7 OVERALL ANNOYANCE/TROUBLE	Never had tinnitus	N
HISTORY ONSET ____	No annoyance	0
	Slight annoyance	1
MIDDLE ____	Moderate annoyance	2
	Severe annoyance	3
RECENT OR END ____	Don't know	D
2.8 INTERFERENCE WITH GETTING	Never had tinnitus	N
TO SLEEP ONSET ____	No	0
	Yes	1
MIDDLE ____	Don't know e.g. due to contamination by sedatives	D
RECENT OR END ____		

2.9 PREVIOUS/EXISTING TINNITUS MANAGEMENT

Codings for 'benefit' column to be used in sections: (2.9.1–2.9.4)

Not applicable N	Moderate benefit 2
None 0	Marked benefit 3
Slight benefit 1	Worse 4
	Don't know D

       Manage Benefit

2.9.1 Medication for tinnitus

_____ _____

_____ _____

_____ _____

Management type codings

Not applicable N	Serc etc 3
None 0	Tegretol 4
Night sedat 1	Tocainide 5
Day sedat/	Uncertain treat-
anti-dep 2	ment 9
Other (state ....) 8	

(if less than 3 used, code others as N)

2.9.2 Ear or body aids or maskers

_____ _____

Not applicable N	Masker 2
None 0	Aid+masker 3
Hearing aid 1	Don't know D

2.9.3 Background maskers (in order of usefulness)

_____ _____

_____ _____

Not applicable N	Clock 2
None 0	Under Pillow 3
Radio or TV 1	Don't know D
Other (state ....) 8	

(if only one used, code other as N)

2.9.4 Other

_____ _____

Not applicable N	Relaxation therapy 2
None 0	Biofeedback 3
Psychiatry 1	Hypnosis 4
Other (state ....) 8	

(if only one used, code other as N)

2.9.5 Member tinnitus association (at any time)

_____

Not applicable N	Don't know D
No 0	Yes 1

2.10 FUTURE MANAGEMENT (patients opinion)

_____

No tinnitus N	Yes, if easy 2
None necessary 0	Yes, will consider
Continue existing 1	anything 3

Assessment of the tinnitus patient

Since the beginnings of recorded history and probably even before that time, mankind has complained about the problem of tinnitus. And yet, oddly enough, tinnitus is not a complaint which is widely or frequently aired by those who suffer from it. The paradox is that tinnitus is very prevalent but remains essentially unknown.

Some luminaries not fearing exposure have made public comment about their tinnitus. Beethoven, in his last will and testament, complains of the irony of the inability to hear outside sounds while at the same time finding it impossible to shut off the inside sounds. Goethe seems to have interpreted his tinnitus as the voice of the Devil punishing him. Bedrich Smetana, most famous for his opera 'The Bartered Bride,' wrote an autobiographic string quartet 'Ma Vlast,' in which '. . . the terrifying high note rings in my ears as a premonition of my cruel fate, that deafness which has now cut me off forever from the blessings of listening to and enjoying our art.' Michelangelo, when commenting upon the ravages of age, complained of the 'racket' in the ears, among other things. Aristotle seems to have been the first to suggest the masking effect of outside sounds upon head noises, implying that he, too, had tinnitus.

In more modern times, Jack Ashley MP, in his book 'Journey into Silence' (The Bodley Head, London, 1973) makes the plague of tinnitus poignantly clear. Ashley describes the ceaseless racket which destroys sleep, prevents concentrating, interrupts mental states, reduces concentration and even retards one's reading ability.

Interestingly enough, most patients find it a simple task to describe what tinnitus does to them, but they find it almost impossible to describe tinnitus itself, and in part, that is why we need presentations on how to assess the tinnitus patient. There is an excessively great variety of kinds and types of tinnitus and if the clinician persists in merely noting whether or not the patient has tinnitus, chaos will continue to reign.

INCIDENCE OF TINNITUS

The National Center for Health Statistics (1967) estimated that there are 36 million American adults with tinnitus in some form. Of that figure, it was further estimated that 20% had tinnitus in a *severe* form. Coles (1981) conducted a survey of England, and came up with a similar proportion of the UK population being affected with tinnitus (see Ch. 3).

These estimates of the high incidence of tinnitus lend weight to the argument that so little effort has been marshalled to combat this problem. We have developed a space effort capable of capturing the uninhabited planets, but we seem unable to direct the effort necessary to conquer that which robs the quality of life for so many.

There is another aspect to the incidence estimates, and that is, that only about 20% of those who have tinnitus have it in its severe form. Later, we will try to describe what severity actually means, but for the present, the clinician should remember that 80% of those patients who list tinnitus as a symptom may need little or no treatment. That is to say, the time and effort afforded those for whom tinnitus is severe is vastly different from that provided to minor cases. If a patient presents with the primary and single complaint of tinnitus, it is likely that the problem is severe, or should be treated as such until proven otherwise. It is also the case when attempting to determine the effectiveness of a given treatment or treatment procedure, that only patients with severe tinnitus should be used as experimental subjects. When the problem is not severe, the need for relief is so reduced as possibly to cause an incorrect interpretation of the value of a given therapy. For example, no patient with minor tinnitus would consider wearing a tinnitus masker, regardless of the effectiveness. The fuss and bother of fitting, adjusting and wearing the masker would produce greater disruption to their lives than that produced by the mild tinnitus itself. Information about the mildness of tinnitus is available in some cases by the ease with which masking is produced. If, for example, masking sounds at 1 or 2 dB above threshold is completely effective in covering the tinnitus, but the patient rejects the masking, we may then assume their tinnitus to be of a relatively mild form.

The American Tinnitus Association, based on the inquiries they receive, has estimated the number of cases of severe tinnitus in the USA to be around 9 million. That estimate is higher than that produced by the Health Survey—20% of 36 million, or 7.2 million. Either estimate, however, leaves us with a very large number of people who need and deserve help. When a new disease appears, we seem very willing to expend considerable effort combating it. For example, in the three years following the advent of acquired immune deficiency (AIDS) disease, the USA alone spent over 4 billion dollars searching for the cause and cure. The incidence of AIDS sufferers is probably 1000 times less than the incidence of tinnitus, and yet properly funded tinnitus research efforts are almost non-existent.

SUBJECTIVE NATURE OF TINNITUS

It is not possible to study that which we cannot measure. Thus, the subjective nature of tinnitus places an added burden upon efforts to study it. Our attempts to measure tinnitus are handicapped by the lack of any objective indicator. Tinnitus does not produce an elevated body temperature, or alterations in blood chemistry, or opacity on X-ray films, or any other presentation which is not under the control of the patient. Since we must rely upon the patient's report, it then becomes necessary to determine the *reliability* of that report. Or, more correctly, we need to design tests for which reliability can be determined. By reliability, we simply mean a consistency of report to a series of retestings. To measure reliability properly, we need to devise tests so that memory of the response cannot operate to provide a false and high-reliability score. This matter of reliability will become clearer a bit later when we discuss pitch-matching schemes.

There are some forms of tinnitus where the demarcation between 'objective' and 'subjective' tinnitus becomes confused. One form of pulsatile or pulsating tinnitus is often judged to be subjective when, in fact, it is not. When the pulsation of the tinnitus is in phase with the heart beat, one should always suspect an objective form of tinnitus and care should be taken to listen for it. Use of a stethoscope in the head and neck region is indicated. If the pulsating tinnitus fluctuates in loudness, then stethoscopic exploration should be conducted during an exacerbated period and these patients should be seen by vascular specialists. (As a brief aside about pulsatile tinnitus, we find that we can almost never effectively mask this kind of tinnitus.)

One more comment about the subjective report of the tinnitus patient. It is important to determine where the tinnitus is located. It is not permissible to assume that the tinnitus is always located in or at the ears. There are cases where it is located at the back of the head, or the top of the head, or it fills the head, or it is to one side of midline, and rarely it is even located outside the head. If the clinician plans to utilize masking as a relief procedure, it is necessary to have the masking sound localized at the same place as the tinnitus. We will explore this concern a bit later in this presentation.

EVALUATION OF THE TINNITUS PATIENT

The assessment of tinnitus patients bears many similarities to the game of bridge. In bridge, no two hands are alike and yet they are sufficiently similar as to allow some general rules of procedure. Those rules, however, do require a liberal use of judgment and often need modification, if not outright violation. To reach an effective management of tinnitus requires a high-level interaction between the clinician and the patient, just as partners must communicate in order to reach a playable contract in bridge. In the game of bridge, communication is always indirectly being effected through a system of 'bidding.' In tinnitus, the communication is indirect, and primarily for the reason that the patient simply does not have command of the necessary language. Indeed, the language available even to the expert for the description of sound is very limited. Thus, the onus for communication between patient and clinician is primarily upon the clinician, he must listen very carefully while resisting the temptation to prejudge.

The plea for quantification of and measurement of tinnitus so that it may be properly represented in medical histories is not new. In 1903, Spalding issued such a plea. Spalding was primarily concerned with the pitch dimension of tinnitus and suggested that different pitch qualities may be related to underlying aetiologies. Since Spalding's time, investigators such as Goodhill (1950), Fowler (1938), Reed (1960), Graham (1965), Hazell (1981a,b), Graham & Newby (1962), etc., have continued to emphasize the need for proper classification of tinnitus. Much of what they have offered by way of assessment we have used, and thus the procedures that have gradually evolved in our clinic are not offered as original contributions. We have borrowed and altered and refined in an almost indiscriminate manner, and the major value we claim for our procedures is that they work and they are based on the experience gained from dealing with over 3000 cases of tinnitus.

Our evaluation of tinnitus patients starts with three questionnaires covering tinnitus, hearing history and general medical history which are mailed to them well in advance of their clinic appointment; they bring the completed questionnaires to the appointment. The questionnaires, which were developed by Mary Meikle, Susan Griest and Nancy Schuff, of our laboratory, are reproduced as Appendixes 4.1, 4.2 and 4.3.

Medical consultation

Prior to coming to our clinic, we require that patients be seen by an otologist or otolaryngologist to ensure that the cause of the tinnitus cannot be medically or surgically corrected. For example, the tinnitus associated with otosclerosis almost always disappears upon completion of successful surgery. Glasgold and Altmann (1966) found tinnitus to be eliminated or greatly reduced in 76% of patients for whom the air-bone gap was closed to within 15 dB or less. Another interesting, but unpursued, observation by Fowler (1944) suggests the possible role of anoxia in tinnitus. He found intravascular agglutination in the vessels of the ocular conjunctiva in a high percentage of patients with continuous tinnitus. Medical examination is necessary to rule out the possibiltigy of VIII nerve tumour. There is also the occasional case where something as simple as wax or hairs or debris on the tympanic membrane can be the culprit. For example, one of our patients who complained of 'clicking' tinnitus was sent to an otolaryngologist to determine the possibility of palatine myoclonus. It turned out that she had a rather large chunk of earwax on the drum which, upon removal, completely relieved the tinnitus. It is surprising that a relatively static affair such as wax on the ear drum was capable of producing a dynamic tinnitus such as 'clicking.'

In tinnitus, however, we have come to believe that almost all things are possible, and these possibilities must be checked prior to proceeding to the non-medical treatment we utilize in our clinic. It is important to remember that tinnitus is a medical problem—it is a symptom associated with pathology of the auditory system—and as such, it must receive medical attention. Once all medical avenues have been explored and the findings are negative, then it is permissible to turn to non-medical approaches in the search for relief.

One final comment about the medical intervention. Not infrequently, and certainly understandably, tinnitus patients will suffer bouts of depression. When this happens, it is common for the patient to be referred to psychiatry, where tricyclic antidepressant medication may well be prescribed. Most of the tricyclic antidepressants list tinnitus as a side effect so that the tinnitus the patient already has may be exacerbated. If this happens, it is usually possible to 'shop around' among the tricyclics until a non-exacerbating one is found for the individual patient. It is also the finding in some few selective cases that tricyclic medications can relieve tinnitus. We have seen three or four patients for whom the tricyclic appears to have broken the cycle, relegating the tinnitus to a minor or inconsequential level.

A recommended procedure for assessing tinnitus patients

The assessment procedure which we wish to recomment is one which has evolved over the years in the Tinnitus Clinic. It is divided into six different processes. They are: 1. Pitch matching (F_T); 2. Loudness matching (LM); 3. Minimum masking level (MML); 4. Test for residual inhibition (RI); 5. Loudness discomfort levels (LDL); and 6. Tests with ear-level equipment.

1. Pitch matching (F_T)

As already indicated, Spalding long ago issued a plea for clinicians to determine the musical notation or pitch of their patients' tinnitus. The method he proposed, however, was somewhat awkward in that it required the physician to play various notes and tones on one or another musical instrument. The patient was to select the tone most like their tinnitus. Spalding's procedure was not unlike that of current-day clinicians who use an audiometer to present various tones from which the patient selects that most resembling their tinnitus. For the most part, this procedure has been used because the clinician has only an audiometer available. The reliability of determining pitch matching (F_T, the frequency corresponding to the pitch of the tinnitus) was investigated in our laboratory. We found considerable variation in a series of test-retests. The subjects for this study were tinnitus patients with tonal tinnitus who claimed that their tinnitus was invariant over time. On the average, these patients selected five different tones as being either 'identical' or 'very close' to their tinnitus. The different tones selected as F_T were clustered toward the middle and high frequencies so that there was never confusion between the tinnitus and low-pitched tones below 1000 Hz. Nevertheless, the precision of identification of F_T was less than desirable.

From this study, several things emerged which have come to help refine pitch matching. For one thing, it became very apparent that patients may easily confuse pitch with loudness, which implies that the loudness of comparison tones should first be set to the same loudness as the tinnitus: then judgments of sameness or difference between comparison stimuli and the tinnitus may be more a matter of pitch than any other quality.

The second thing we stumbled onto was the matter of 'octave confusion.' Not infrequently, patients will select a given test tone as being very close or identical to their tinnitus when, in fact, it is one octave below the correct identification. A random selection of 50 patients from our clinic was surveyed for octave confusion. Twenty-four patients did not receive the octave confusion test for the following reasons: some had a noise-type tinnitus, some had 'crickets', for some the pitch identification was too high to allow testing at an octave above it, and some had high-frequency hearing losses of sufficient magnitude to preclude octave confusion testing. Of the 26 remaining patients, 3 presented unclear results, 7 revealed no octave confusion, and 16 did reveal octave confusion. These data suggest that about 62% of the time, octave confusion reigns and furthermore, that such confusion could cause a serious pitch misidentification for patients' tinnitus. Thus, it has become necessary to install a check for octave confusion in the pitch-matching test.

A variety of procedures were tried in an effort to obtain the most reliable pitch matches possible. From this effort, there emerged the Two-Alternative Forced-Choice procedure. This procedure involves the sequential presentation of two tones requiring the patient to indicate which tone is more like their tinnitus. Presentations may be repeated upon patient demand. Prior to sequential presentations, each tone is established at the same loudness as the tinnitus. The test tones can be selected according to a variety of schemes, depending upon the demands of the study or purpose at hand. In the clinic situation, we routinely select a series of tones starting at 100 Hz and proceeding upward in 100 Hz increments. Table 4.1 shows how a typical series might be represented.

Table 4.1 Pitch matching: typical patient's response

Trial no.	Comparison tones, Hz	Response, Hz
1	1000 vs. 2000	2000
2	2000 vs. 3000	3000
3	3000 vs. 4000	4000
4	4000 vs. 5000	5000
5	5000 vs. 6000	5000

At Trial 5, we seem to have run past the F_T area, in that 5000 Hz was selected over 6000 Hz. At this point, it is essential to conduct the test for octave confusion, which in this example, would compare 5000 Hz with 10 000 Hz. Not infrequently, the patient will select the higher frequency, which in this case would be 10 000 Hz. Consider what has happened here. The patient consistently selected the higher of the two presentations until 5000 Hz was paired with 6000 Hz, at which time the lower frequency was selected, implying that a precise pitch match is below 6000 Hz and possibly above 5000 Hz, when in fact the best match in this case may be well above 6000 Hz if there is octave confusion. Each clinician is encouraged to listen to octave pairs presented sequentially and where each is established at a sensation level of about 5 dB. Such a demonstration easily reveals how patients can come to make the octave confusion.

The Two-Alternative Forced-Choice procedure for pitch matching was tested for its reliability using a multiple test-retest situation distributed over a matter of weeks. There were some errors but on the average the patients selected only *two* frequencies which they classed as identical or close to their tinnitus. These two selections were never separated by more than the established increment between stimuli which was 1000 Hz.

In a study of 1800 tinnitus patients, Meikle and Walsh (1984) found that 54% of the patients matched their tinnitus to tones above 3000 Hz; 30% were from 3000 to 5000 Hz; 19% were from 5000 to 9000 Hz; 4% were from 9000 to 11 000 Hz and 1% from 11 000 to 15 000 Hz. In addition, 21% were from 1000 to 3000 Hz and 11% were below 1000 Hz. In trying to do pitch matching with tinnitus patients, it is probably worth remembering that Meikle and Walsh found 89% matched the pitch of their tinnitus to tones above 1000 Hz. It seems reasonable to conclude that more than 11% of the cases have low frequency tinnitus, but most likely, many of these cases are truly minor and consequently do not show up in our clinic.

As one reviews the pitch-matching data from tinnitus patients, it seems to be in sharp contrast to what we know about the human's ability for pitch discrimination. The normal human ear is capable of extreme sensitivity in discriminating differences in pitch. Is it the fact that 90% of tinnitus patients do not have normal ears that makes their ability to match pitch far below expectation? It certainly seems reasonable that the presence of a damaged ear should have an influence on pitch matching but there is something more. Tests of pitch discrimination (and note that I have equated pitch discrimination and tinnitus pitch matching) are usually done at intensity levels well above threshold, such as at sensation levels of 40 dB or more. Pitch discrimination ability declines as the intensity levels are reduced. We conducted a little demonstration of this point, using laboratory personnel who possessed not only normal hearing but also considerable knowledge about sound. Our procedure was to establish an artificial 'tinnitus' in one ear of each subject ($n=9$), high-pitched tone (7000 or 8000 or 9000 Hz) at a sensation level of 10 dB. Next, a series of tones (also at 10 dB SL) were presented to the opposite ear and each subject was required to judge whether or not each tone was the same as, or different from, their 'tinnitus'. Only one subject performed correctly; she was also the only subject with a knowledge of music. The record for the other eight subjects was utter chaos – not only did they identify many incorrect tones as being identical to their tinnitus, but they also classed the correct match as being very different. From all this, we concluded that the low-intensity level or the low loudness level of the tinnitus (see below) makes pitch matching a difficult task under the best of circumstances.

One final consideration about tinnitus pitch matching. We seem to find that a fairly large percentage of our patients possess what can best be classified as tonal tinnitus. If the tinnitus is truly tonal, does that mean that a properly-tuned external tone would produce a beating interaction? Wegel (1931) claims to have obtained beats with his own tinnitus and an external tone. Davis et al (1946) attempted to detect beats between noise-induced tinnitus and an exploring tone and were successful in only one of the five cases tested. Davis later (1951) expressed doubts about Wegel's claim. Lackner (1976) claims that tinnitus induced by head injury is tonal and can produce beats with external exploring tones. In our clinic, 100 patients with tonal tinnitus were explored for the production of beats and only four cases were found. These findings suggest to us that tonal tinnitus for the most part is not a pure tone, but probably a very narrow band of noise which is primarily tonal in nature. In a simulated situation it is almost impossible to produce 'beats' between two narrow bands of noise centered at the same frequency, for the reason that the noise is relatively unstable.

A few final comments as to attempting to duplicate or determine the pitch quality of tinnitus. Some patients complain of 'crickets' and this condition can be reproduced by the simultaneous presentation of two tones. The frequency region of these two tones is between 1000 Hz and 7000 Hz, although the most frequent matches are in the 3000 and 4000 Hz region. In this region, the separation between the two tones is 60 or 70 Hz. A simultaneous presentation of 3000 and 3060 Hz produces a clear and good 'cricket' effect. Using tones in the 4000 Hz region requires about a 70 Hz separation for a good 'cricket' effect. With the dual simultaneous presentation, the patient can quickly indicate whether the overall pitch needs raising or lowering.

Some patients experience a noise-type tinnitus which in Reed's (1960) study accounted for 35% of the cases. We find a higher proportion of tonal cases, but there is a substantial number of noise-type cases. Most of these cases have what the patient terms 'a hissing' which means a pitch-pitched band of noise. Attempts to duplicate a noise-type tinnitus is difficult and frequently depends upon the steepness of the skirts on either side of the band of noise. Use of a tunable noise generator can, in most cases, give a reasonable estimate of the approximate pitch region of the patient's tinnitus, especially if the comparison presentations are kept to the loudness level of the tinnitus.

There are some cases of highly complex tinnitus which defy duplication: for example, Meikle and Whitney (1984) surveyed 1514 cases, finding 28 ($>2\%$) for whom five different sounds constituted their tinnitus; to duplicate such complex tinnitus accurately would be nearly impossible. About the only hope would be by the procedure of Hazell (1979, 1981a,b) which utilizes an electronics music synthesizer.

In the survey by Meikle and Whitney (1984) of 854 patients, 453 (53%) claimed a tonal tinnitus, 56 (6%) indicated 'crickets', 152 (18%) indicated hissing, 102 (12%) were 'whistle' or 'steam whistle'; thus some 89% of the cases can be expected to perform reasonably well on pitch matching procedures. In the typical clinical setting using a tinnitus synthesizer, it should be possible to effect fairly accurate pitch matching within 15 minutes or so.

2. Loudness matching (LM)

It is almost automatic for the uninitiated to assume that tinnitus is severe when it is loud. That would undoubtedly be the case, but the fact is that tinnitus is not loud. Fowler (1942) was the first to point out that tinnitus, when matched to the intensity of an external sound, has a sensation level of only about 5–10 dB. In contrast to most of our daily ambient environmental sounds, a sensation at 5–10 dB is indeed low. The findings of Fowler were confirmed by Reed (1960), Vernon (1976) and Goodwin and Johnson (1980).

Keep in mind that the Chinese torture of antiquity was not to hit the head with a hard blow, but merely to arrange for a drop of water to repeatedly fall on the forehead, which presumably led to insanity. Tinnitus is much like the Chinese torture. It is not loud, but it is constant and inescapable.

Perhaps the unremitting constancy of tinnitus produces its severity. According to a survey of 1068 tinnitus patients by Meikle and Walsh (1984) where patients rated the severity of their tinnitus on a 10-point scale, it was possible to break the ratings into 'mild,' 'moderate,' or 'severe.' Ratings of 1 to 4 were classed as mild and found in 8% of the cases, ratings of 5 through 8 were classed moderate and were found in 70% of the cases, ratings of 9 through 10 were classed as severe and were found in 22% of the cases.

Our purpose here is to discuss tinnitus loudness matching, and not the topic of severity. Nevertheless, it is of interest that the question as to what correlates with severity has not been answered, despite studies of the obvious leads. To pursue the topic further, see the work by Meikle & Walsh (1984).

We have adopted a standardized procedure for the measurement of loudness of tinnitus. Most of the data can be obtained from the pitch matching procedures, since all stimuli used there were first established at the same loudness as the tinnitus.

We only use an ascending intensity series, because a descending series could produce residual inhibition, which in turn would provide a spuriously low estimate of the loudness of tinnitus. Typically, we start with a 1000 Hz tone as a subthreshold level and increase the intensity in 2 dB increments until threshold for that tone is reached. This threshold value is recorded. Next, the intensity is increased in 1 dB increments until the loudness of the comparison tone is equal to that of the tinnitus, and that level is recorded. The difference between these two values is taken as the loudness of the tinnitus in sensation level. A typical data sheet for loudness matching is given as Table 4.2.

Table 4.2 Typical loudness matching data sheet

Stimulus, Hz	Threshold	Loudness match	Sensation level, dB
1000	20	42	22
2000	30	48	18
3000	50	61	11
4000	65	72	7
▸5000	60	65	5
6000	50	55	5
7000	45	50	5

Position of arrow indicates F_T

The tinnitus in this case was located at 5000 Hz and note that the loudness estimates progressively declined as the comparison tones came closer to F_T. In another source (Vernon & Meikle 1981), we referred to this as a converging loudness function or a decreasing loudness function, where the loudness function is strongly dependent upon the frequency of the comparison tones. Note that the loudness match reaches a minimum at or near the tinnitus frequency (F_T). At frequencies above F_T, the loudness level may increase again or remain at the minimum level.

A second form of loudness function seen in our clinic is a constant function which is independent of frequency. If, for example, the loudness match at F_T is, say, 5 dB SL (sensation level), then it will also be 5 dB SL at any frequency used as a comparison tone.

Except in those cases of unilateral severe hearing loss, the loudness matching can be conducted either ipsilaterally or contralaterally. As a general rule, we tend to use contralateral presentations unless the patient requests otherwise, which is rarely the case.

In the survey of 502 tinnitus patients conduced by Meikle and Walsh (1984), 51% of the patients matched the loudness of their tinnitus at F_T at 0–3 dB SL, 28% from 4 to 6 dB SL, 8% at 7–9 dB SL, and 11% above 10 dB. These data indicate that 79% of tinnitus patients have tinnitus at a loudness of 6 dB SL or less, and yet these same patients have presented to our clinic with the primary complaint of tinnitus. It is unfortunate that in one of the earlier works on tinnitus, Fowler (1942) instructed physicians and clinicians to use the loudness data to convince their patients they did not have a serious problem. To this day, that attitude persists in the minds of many of the professionals encountered by tinnitus patients, and it is small wonder that they often seek help from a large number of professionals.

A final comment about the loudness of tinnitus. It may be that we are measuring loudness incorrectly and/or we have missed some fundamental aspect of this phenomenon. The work of Goodwin & Johnson (1980) emphasizes the possible role of recruitment and it seems reasonable to conclude that recruitment can, at least in part, make a given loudness level of tinnitus appear more intense. Recruitment, however, does not seem to explain the whole situation. How, for example, can the quality of life be destroyed by the presence of a 3 dB SL sound? Even if, via recruitment, it is more nearly a 6 dB or 12 dB sound. Something is wrong here and I am persuaded that we have missed something, but what is it? Is tinnitus a faulty inhibition system? In so many patients, tinnitus does not behave like external sounds; instead it seems to have some sort of direct input or a pre-empted awareness that makes its presence known in a manner different from ordinary auditory perception. There is need here to study patients for whom the tinnitus fluctuates widely. Would their loudness matches be the same during 'good phases' as during 'bad phases'? If they have a 3 dB SL match during bad phases it is hard to imagine that reducing to 2 dB or 1 dB or 0 dB would constitute a good phase. It may turn out that measures of the loudness of tinnitus bear no relationship to the perceived severity of tinnitus, but we need to know that, otherwise we will tend to conclude that we are measuring loudness incorrectly.

3. *Minimum masking level* (MML)

If one is involved in a tinnitus clinic which offers masking as a relief procedure, the need for a determination of MML is obvious. Aside from that, however, information about MML will provide an additional evaluation to be used for the testing of various potential relief procedures. For example, consider the case for tocainide. Tocainide is a near-oral analogue of lidocaine. Intravenous lidocaine has a suppression effect upon a high percentage of tinnitus patients (see Goodey 1981, Israel et al 1982, Melding et al 1978, Shea & Harrell 1978 and Lewy 1937 for an introduction to this challenging topic in tinnitus research; also Ch. 10).

Relief is produced by lidocaine in a large majority of patients. Unfortunately, however, it is short-lasting, usually less than half an hour. Thus, an intravenous procedure which would require many repetitions is not a practical affair. Nevertheless, lidocaine offers a ray of hope and the development of tocainide as an oral analogue of lidocaine (or nearly so) was viewed with high optimism for tinnitus. The resulting tests of tocainide have turned out to be very disappointing. There is, however, a possibility that tocainide plus masking may offer relief as has been suggested by Goodey (1981). Thus, knowledge of the maskability of tinnitus may provide evaluative information about tinnitus which is important for a variety of considerations.

The question when considering masking concerns the nature of the masking sound. What kind of sound or sounds should be used as the most effective masker?

One thing we do know and that is that white noise is not an appropriate masking noise for tinnitus. For tinnitus patients with a hearing loss (90% in our clinic) (Vernon 1978), a wide-band noise such as white noise will excessively stimulate the normal or near-normal non-tinnitus portion of the hearing well in advance of masking the tinnitus. Moreover, Penner et al (1981) have demonstrated that with white noise there is an adaptation to the masking effect so that the tinnitus requires progressively more and more sound in order to effect masking. For a report on the successful use of masking to relieve tinnitus, see Vernon (1982), Schleuning et al (1980) and Vernon (1978, 1979).

We have elected to use two kinds of masking sounds: a band of noise from 3000 Hz through 12 000 Hz (recall that, according to Meikle & Walsh (1984), 54% of our cases have tinnitus above 3000 Hz), and a tone located at the tinnitus frequency.

In a typical situation, we determine MML for the ipsilateral ear, or in the bilateral case for each ear independently. An ascending series of increasing intensities is always used so as to minimize the possibility of residual inhibition. In two different surveys in our clinic (Vernon 1978, Meikle & Walsh 1984) the incidence of bilateral tinnitus was nearly the same. About 63% of patients have bilateral tinnitus and in such cases one should constantly check to see if contralateral masking can be effected.

In the usual case, the masking sound is increased from a subliminal level to the point of detection. At this threshold intensity, the patient is asked if they can hear their tinnitus in the ipsilateral ear. If the response is positive, the masking sound is turned off, then its intensity is increased by 2 dB and it is re-presented. The masking intensity is increased in this manner by 2 dB increments until the patient is confident they cannot hear their tinnitus in the ipsilateral ear in the presence of the masking sound and this level is recorded as the MML. In the case of bilateral tinnitus, the clinician must constantly remind the patient that only the ipsilateral ear is of concern. There are also some few cases where the patient does not realize that they have bilateral tinnitus so that they continue to report the presence of their tinnitus long after the ipsilateral side has been completely masked. A bit of training and a lot of patience is in order for some cases.

Once the MML has been determined for a given ear in the bilateral cases, we always ask if any masking has been effected in the contralateral ear, and record the result. Recently, we surveyed 291 cases of MML determinations, of which 53 (18%) revealed some degree of contralateral masking. Of thosle cases displaying contralateral masking, the masking effect was complete in 32 cases (60%) and partial in the remainder. Information of this sort is often useful in planning the best strategy for a relief programme.

Why use a pure tone as the masking sound to determine MML? We do this only to get some idea as to how restrictive the masking sound needs to be in order to produce the most effective masking. If the MML turns out to be vastly different using a band of noise instead of the pure tone at F_T, it may suggest incorrect identification of F_T or it may suggest a particular manner by which to effect masking. As a rule of thumb, if MML turns out to be 20 dB SL or more, then use of a masking programme is doubtful (see also Ch. 5).

Masking of tinnitus when the localization of tinnitus is in the head. There is one unusual case we have encountered in our clinic which requires special attention: tinnitus which is localized at or near the centre of the head. This situation came to our attention in cases where masking was found to be easily effected for the patient using the tinnitus synthesizer under earphones, but, oddly enough, was not possible at all using ear-level equipment. The solution to this situation was the difference in the masking sounds generated by the tinnitus synthesizer and those generated by ear level equipment. In the synthesizer there is a single noise generator, the output of which is split into two branches, so that when bilateral stimulation is used an identical sound goes to the two ears. Such stimulation causes the masking sound to be localized in the middle of the head and thus masks the tinnitus which is also located in the middle of the head. With the ear-level tinnitus maskers or tinnitus instruments, two different noise generators are employed, with the result that non-coherent sound is supplied to the two ears. Moreover, this kind of sound stimulation causes the patient to perceive the masking sound at each ear and not in the head, so that they now hear three sounds. We have come to believe that in order to mask tinnitus properly, the masking sound must be perceived at the same location as the tinnitus. Thus, it behoves us carefully to question the perceived location of the tinnitus.

Once again, we see yet another difference between tinnitus and physical sound. Identical sound simultaneously delivered to the two ears causes a midline in-the-head localization of a single sound. How can it be the case that some patients complain of identical tinnitus sounds which are located, not in the head, but at the two ears, and perceived as two distinct and separate but identical sounds?

The measurement of MMLs must take into account the localization of the tinnitus being masked. And the same consideration is essential when one attempts to effect a masking programme. Unfortunately at present we have no ear-level equipment capable of delivering coherent masking to the two ears. Something of a variation on a Bi-Cros arrangement is needed. For a few patients, we have used the Sony Walkman with a cassette tape recording of the masking noise found to be most appropriate for the given patient. We selected the Sony Walkman because its frequency response goes well up into the high-frequency region so often needed.

4. Residual inhibition (RI)

Residual ihibition is defined as the suppression or complete elimination of tinnitus for a temporary period following masking. This phenomenon has been known since the work of Spalding in 1903. The term 'Residual Inhibition' was coined by Vernon (1977) to honour Feldmann's (1971) work on masking of tinnitus. Feldmann stated that the interaction of external sounds upon tinnitus was not a true case of masking, rather, he argued, it is more like an *inhibition*. We agreed with Feldmann, but had already introduced the term 'masking' to describe the action of the tinnitus masker and since the term 'tinnitus masker' was established, it was too late to change. Perhaps it was an inadequate gesture, but our attempt to display agreement with Feldmann was to invent the term 'residual inhibition'.

Residual inhibition comes in many forms, but it is not an inconsequential or capricious affair: in one form or another, it is found in 88% of the patients attending our clinic. That it is so prevalent causes us to claim that the ultimate explanation of those mechanisms underlying tinnitus must also explain residual inhibition, for it is an integral part of tinnitus (see Vernon 1981).

Our test for residual inhibition is as follows. Using a band of noise (3000–12 000 Hz) which is established at MML +10 dB for 60 s, the duration of the resulting residual inhibition is measured (the quantities +10 dB and 60 s are arbitrary selections). We wanted to increase the intensity of the masking sound to enhance the production of residual inhibition; at the same time, we did not want to make it uncomfortable for the patient. We wanted to present the masking sound long enough to permit the production of residual inhibition, but not so long as to bore the patient. Recently we studied the effect of increasing the intensity of the masking sound and found that the duration of residual inhibition was unrelated to the various masking levels we used. The magnitude or the degree of suppression seem to be positively related to the intensity of the masking sound.

As indicated, residual inhibition comes in a variety of forms and without going into a description of these kinds, it nevertheless should be indicated that a given patient is reliable: i.e. on test-retest his or her form of residual inhibition is consistent.

Residual inhibition can play a role in the use of masking for relief of tinnitus. For the most part, the lower the intensity of the masking sound (while still effectively covering the tinnitus), the more readily it is accepted as a substitute for the tinnitus. Always keep in mind that masking, in any of its forms, is only a substitution of an external sound for the internal one. Thus it follows that if, because of residual inhibition, the patient can systematically reduce the level of the masker while still obtaining relief, it is not only more likely to be acceptable but also more easily ignored.

There are two major forms of residual inhibition which should be indicated in the clinical tests. Some cases find a temporary total absence of tinnitus after masking and this is termed Complete Residual Inhibition (CRI). If a patient goes into CRI, after about 30 seconds or so, they will notice the faint reappearance of the tinnitus which gradually, or in some specific fashion, increases until it returns to its customary level. The return function is designated as Partial Residual Inhibition (PRI). It, too, often lasts only about 30 seconds. In some cases, only PRI is obtained. Intersubject variation in magnitude and duration of RI is considerable. A survey of 63 patients by Vernon & Meikle (1981) revealed a few who experienced CRI for over five minutes after only one minute of masking. That survey also showed that the majority of patients displaying either CRI or PRI do so for less than one minute.

Needless to say, the reports of patients who have experienced extensive and profound residual inhibition after long periods of masking prompt us to search for ways to improve residual inhibition. To date, despite concerted efforts, we do not know how to prolong this effect. There are, however, several intruiguing items. Residual inhibition is never observed when using hearing aids only to mask the tinnitus. In about 10% of the cases, it is possible to completely mask out the tinnitus with use of hearing aids alone. But these patients never experience residual inhibition; does that mean that ambient environmental sounds are ineffectual masking sounds? Or is their non-continuous nature at fault? Another interesting point involves bilateral masking produced by a unilateral masker. In such cases, it is rare to obtain contralateral residual inhibition.

During periods of induced residual inhibition, we have searched for alterations in the threshold sensitivity at the tinnitus frequency. Using 50 patients as subjects, we find a slight but consistent decrease in threshold sensitivity at F_T. It is unlikely that this decrease in sensitivity is any more than a typical temporary threshold shift (TTS). TTS, however, is not residual inhibition, since the time course of recovery is different in the two cases.

For the present, we find this topic of residual inhibition to be a confusing affair. On test-retest it is reliably present, indicating that the phenomenon is real, but beyond that we do not know what factors influence it. We use RI as a way of instructing patients about masking, but we do not understand it. Clearly, this intriguing aspect of tinnitus merits concerted research efforts.

5. Loudness discomfort levels (LDL)

Recently, Tyler & Conrad-Armes (1983) devised a measure which has promise as a possible indicator of the perceived severity of tinnitus. We have slightly modified this procedure and have just initiated the LDL measures. The idea is to determine how well sound is tolerated in the frequency region of the tinnitus, compared to the same measure in the non-tinnitus and more normal hearing region.

A tone located at F_T is increased in the tinnitus ear or ears until the threshold of detection is reached. The tone is then increased in 2 dB increments until the loudness discomfort level is reached. It is well known that LDL is easily influenced by the instructions. Our instruction will be: 'Assume this sound is the level of your radio or television set. Indicate the minimum loudness level at which you would turn the set down.'

The LDL is determined not only for F_T but also in the highest normal or nearly normal hearing region, using a tone at a frequency appropriate for that region. It is likely that tolerance for loudness at F_T is truncated as compared to other non-tinnitus hearing areas which may be either normal or impaired regions.

6. Acute trials with ear level equipment

Upon completion of the clinic testing, the patient is given an opportunity to experience a variety of masking devices first-hand. Since most patients have hearing losses, our first attempt to relieve the tinnitus is by use of hearing aids alone. That procedure is appropriate in less than 10% of the cases, but when it works, we usually go no further and recommend the fitting of hearing aids.

When hearing aids alone do not work, we then explain masking to the patient, emphasizing that they, not us, will determine whether or not masking is appropriate.

The typical case is the patient with high-frequency bilateral hearing loss and high-frequency bilateral tinnitus. In such cases, we fit tinnitus instruments (a combination masker and hearing aid) such as the Audiotone TA-641 or the Starkey MA-3. First, the amplification is adjusted to the proper level for the patient; it is essential that this be done properly before adding the masking sound. Then and only then is the masking sound added in small increments, finding the minimum level at which the tinnitus is covered up. In the majority of cases where masking is successful, the masking level is very low, being established at threshold or only slightly above it. When it is necessary to adjust the masking level well above threshold, it is likely that the patient will not find masking to be an acceptable substitute for their tinnitus. We make a special point of being sure that the patient understands the goal of masking, based on the concept of substitution, and we make it clear that masking under the best of conditions is *not a cure*—it is only a relief procedure. We try a variety of masking units—tinnitus instrument or tinnitus maskers—on each patient, so that they can select from among the available masking sounds.

One puzzling and interesting thing has occurred. The tinnitus instrument has an internal adjustment for low-frequency, mid-frequency and high-frequency hearing loss, one would assume that best results would be obtained by using the internal high-frequency setting. Just the opposite is the case—most do best with the setting on low-frequency emphasis. The moral here seems to be: TRY ALL PERMUTATIONS OF ALL PARAMETERS BEFORE SURRENDER.

Failure to use the tinnitus instrument (UK: combination instrument) has been a common mistake we have seen in other clinics. The failure to use bilateral equipment is another common mistake. Where appropriate, we insist upon use of bilateral equipment from the beginning, rather than starting with a unilateral fitting and later adding the second unit. All too often the only appropriate procedure is a bilateral one and to do anything less is to discourage the patient.

Final instructions to patients

We find that even the procedures which are most obvious to us are not necessarily obvious to tinnitus patients. They need to be told to use masking only when they need it and that they must work out a schedule which works best for them.

We instruct *all* patients to avoid *all* loud sounds. One of the easiest ways to exacerbate tinnitus, regardless of aetiology, is by exposure to loud sounds. Use of caffeine can also exacerbate tinnitus for some cases. Thus patients are encouraged to abstain from caffeine for one month to determine its effect on their tinnitus. Cautions about the use of aspirin are issued and all patients are instructed to avoid all forms of marijuana. Finally, the patients for whom masking devices are recommended are instructed to report back to the clinic one month after being fitted with their device.

SUMMARY

A review of the assessment procedures which we consider to be necessary for each tinnitus patient is as follows:

1. *Otological evaluation.* Each patient should have a thorough otological examination prior to other tests in order to determine the presence and extent of medical involvement.

2. *Audiological testing.* Routine audiological evaluation is needed to determine the hearing capability of each patient. In some cases, special audiological tests may be indicated.
3. *Tinnitus testing.* To quantify the tinnitus, the following tests are conducted:
   a. pitch match of the tinnitus (FT)
   b. loudness match (LM)
   c. minimum masking level (MML)
   d. tests for residual inhibition (RI)
   e. loudness discomfort levels (LDL)
4. *Recommendations for relief.* In our particular clinic, ear-level masking devices of various sorts are tried to determine whether or not masking is able to provide relief and if so, which device best provides that service.

REFERENCES

Coles R R A 1981 Epidemiology of tinnitus. In: Evered D, Lawrenson G (eds) Tinnitus. Ciba Foundation Symposium 85, Pitman, London
Davis H 1951 Psychophysiology of hearing and deafness. In: Stevens S S (ed) Handbook of Experimental Psychology. Wiley, New York
Davis H, Morga C T, Hawkins J E, Galambos R, Smith F W 1946 Temporary deafness following exposure to loud tones and noise. Laryngoscope 56: 19–21
Feldmann H 1971 Homolateral and contralateral masking of tinnitus by noise bands and by pure tones. Audiology 10: 138–144
Fowler E P 1938 New methods for accurately determining the threshold of bone conduction and for measuring tinnitus and its effect upon obstruction and neural deafness. Transactions of the American Otologic Society 26: 154–171
Fowler E P 1942 The 'illusion of loudness' of tinnitus: Its etiology and treatment. Laryngoscope 52: 275–285
Fowler E P 1944 Head noises in normal and in disordered ears: Significance, measurement, differentiation and treatment. Archives of Otolaryngology 39: 498–503
Glasgold A, Altmann F 1966 The effect of stapes surgery on tinnitus in otosclerosis. Laryngoscope 76: 1524–1532
Goodey R J 1981 Drugs in the treatment of tinnitus. In: Evered D, Lawrenson G (eds) Tinnitus. Ciba Foundation Symposium 85, Pitman, London pp 263–272
Goodhill V 1950 The management of tinnitus. Laryngoscope 60: 442–450
Goodwin P E, Johnson R M 1980 A comparison of reaction times to tinnitus and nontinnitus frequencies. Ear and Hearing 1: 148–155
Graham J T, Newby H A 1962 Acoustical characteristics of tinnitus. Archives of Otolaryngology 75: 162–167
Graham J T 1965 Tinnitus aurium. Acta Otolaryngologica Supplement 202: 1–32
Hazell J W P 1979 Tinnitus. British Journal of Hospital Medicine 22: 468–471
Hazell J W P 1981a Measurement of tinnitus in humans. In: Evered D, Lawrenson G (eds) Tinnitus. Ciba Foundation Symposium 85, Pitman, London, pp 35–48
Hazell J W P 1981b Patterns of Tinnitus: Medical audiologic findings. In: Shulman A (ed) Tinnitus: Proceedings of the First International Tinnitus Seminar, New York 1979. Journal of Laryngology and Otology Supplement 4: 39–47
Israel J M, Connelly J S, McTigue S T, Brummett R E, Brown J D 1982 Lidocaine in the treatment of tinnitus aurium. Archives of Otolaryngology 108: 471–473
Lackner J R 1976 The auditory characteristics of tinnitus resulting from cerebral injury. Experimental Neurology 51: 54–67
Lewy R B 1937 Treatment of tinnitus aurium by intravenous use of local anaesthetic agents. Archives of Otolaryngology 25: 178–183

Meikle M B, Walsh E T 1984 Characteristics of tinnitus and related observations in over 1800 tinnitus clinic patients. In: Shulman A (ed) Proceedings of the Second International Tinnitus Seminar, Journal of Laryngology and Otology Supplement 9: 17–21

Meikle M B, Whitney S 1984 Computer-assisted analysis of reported tinnitus sounds. In: Shulman A (ed) Proceedings of the Second International Tinnitus Seminar, New York 1983. Journal of Laryngology and Otology Supplement 9: 188–192

Melding P S, Goodey R J, Thorne P R 1978 The use of intravenous lignocaine in the diagnosis and treatment of tinnitus. Journal of Laryngology and Otology 92: 115–121

National Center for Health Statistics 1967 Hearing levels of adults by race, region and area of residence. United States 1960–1962. US Dept of Health, Education & Welfare Vital and Health Statistics Publication Series 11, No. 26. Washington, US Government Printing Office, Hyattsville Maryland

Penner M J, Brauth S, Hood L 1981 The temporal course of the masking of tinnitus as a basis for inferring its origin. Journal of Speech and Hearing Research 24: 257–261

Reed G F 1960 An audiometric study of 200 cases of subjective tinnitus. Archives of Otolaryngology 71: 84–94

Schleuning A J, Johnson R M, Vernon J A 1980 Evaluation of a tinnitus masking program: A follow-up study of 598 patients. Ear and Hearing 1: 71–74

Shea J J, Harell M 1978 Management of tinnitus aurium with lidocaine and carbamazepine. Laryngoscope 88: 1477–1484

Spalding J A 1903 Tinnitus: With a plea for its more accurate musical notation. Archives of Otolaryngology 32: 263–272

Tyler R S, Conrad-Armes D 1983 The determination of tinnitus loudness considering the effects of recruitment. Journal of Speech and Hearing Research 26: 59–72

Vernon J A 1976 The loudness (?) of tinnitus. Speech and Hearing Action 44: 17–19

Vernon J A 1977 Attempts to relieve tinnitus. Journal of the American Audiology Society 2: 124–131

Vernon J A 1978 Information from UOHSC Tinnitus Clinic. American Tinnitus Association Newsletter 3: 1–4

Vernon J A 1979 The use of masking for relief of tinnitus. In: Silverstein H, Norrell H (eds) Neurological surgery of the ear, Vol. 2. Aesculapius, Birmingham, Alabama, pp 104–118

Vernon J A 1981 Some observations on residual inhibition. In: Paparella M M, Meyerhoff W L (eds) Sensorineural hearing loss, vertigo & tinnitus, Williams and Wilkins, Baltimore, pp 138–143

Vernon J A 1982 Relief of tinnitus by masking treatment. In: English G M (ed) Otolaryngology. Harper and Row, Philadelphia

Vernon J A, Meikle M B 1981 Tinnitus masking: Unresolved problems. In: Evered D, Lawrenson G (eds) Tinnitus. Ciba Foundation Symposium 85, Pitman, London, pp 239–256

Wegel R L 1931 A study of tinnitus. Archives of Otolaryngology 14: 158–165

APPENDIX 4.1

Tinnitus clinic questionnaire: Tinnitus

Name _____ Age _____ Birthdate _____
     Last   First   Initial

Address _____

                                                        Telephone _____
     City   State   Zip Code

Referred to tinnitus clinic by _____

1. How long have you been aware of *tinnitus* (noises or sounds in your ears or head)?

2. Were illness, accident or other special circumstances associated with the onset of your tinnitus?

                            Please explain briefly

3. Where does your tinnitus appear to be located?

   Where is it worst? (if in more than one location)

4. Has the location of your tinnitus changed since it first began?   NO   YES

   Describe briefly

5. Since it started, has your tinnitus

       grown worse   remained about the same   improved

6. At present, is your tinnitus constantly there, or do you hear it only part of the time?

              CONSTANTLY THERE   HEAR IT ONLY PART OF THE TIME

   If you hear your tinnitus only part of the time, describe briefly how much of the time it is there

7. Does your tinnitus usually sound similar to any of the following?
   (Check all that apply to your tinnitus)

Ringing	Hissing	Sizzling	Pulsating
Clear tone	Buzzing	Transformer noise	Pounding
More than one tone	Hum	High tension wire	Ocean roar
Whistle	Music	Crickets	Clicking

   Other _____
                           Describe

8. Has your tinnitus always sounded like question 7, or have you noticed changes in the type of sound heard?

         THE TYPE OF SOUND HAS STAYED ABOUT THE SAME
         THE TYPE OF SOUND HAS CHANGED AS FOLLOWS

9. About how long has your tinnitus sounded the way it does now?

Tinnitus Strength or Loudness

10. How would you describe the strength or loudness of your *usual* tinnitus?

0	Absent	3	Very intense
1	Barely noticeable	4	Uncomfortably intense
2	Moderate		

11. Since it first started, has your tinnitus grown any louder or softer?

    NO, NO SIGNIFICANT CHANGE   YES
                                              (Describe changes)

12. Does the loudness of your tinnitus tend to fluctuate (sometimes louder, sometimes softer)?

    NO   YES

    If yes, how often do changes occur?

    When do you usually notice changes?

    How large are the changes usually?   Barely noticeable
                                                Moderate
                                                Very marked
                                                Unpredictable

Tinnitus Severity

13. Does your tinnitus interfere with sleep?   NO   YES   SOMETIMES

14. Do you feel tinnitus has caused you significant problems in any of the following ways?

Makes you feel irritable or nervous	NO	YES	SOMETIMES
Makes you feel tired or ill	NO	YES	SOMETIMES
Makes it difficult to relax	NO	YES	SOMETIMES

15. Has tinnitus caused you any of the following problems

	At work	In leisure time
Made it uncomfortable to be in quiet		
Made it difficult to concentrate		
Made it harder to interact pleasantly with others		

16. a. Are there any other problems tinnitus has caused you in your work life?

    NO   YES   If yes, describe

    b. Have you changed jobs because of tinnitus   NO   YES

    If yes, explain what changes you made

17. a. How would you rate the severity of your tinnitus (check more than one level if needed)?

1	Tinnitus is there if attended to but it is not very irritating and can usually be ignored
2	Tinnitus is often irritating but can be ignored much of the time
3	Tinnitus difficult to ignore even with effort
4	Tinnitus is always present at an irritating level – often causes considerable distress
5	Tinnitus is more than irritating, causes an overwhelming problem much or all of the time

b. How would you rate the degree to which tinnitus interferes with your life?
(Check more than one level if needed)

1   Tinnitus causes little or no interference with work or social activities
2   Tinnitus causes some interference, but I can live with it
3   Because of tinnitus, it takes considerable effort to maintain normal work or social activities
4   Tinnitus is serious interference with normal lifestyle—can do only simple tasks
5   Tinnitus renders me unable to perform any work or social activities

18. Do you feel that the severity of your tinnitus varies from time to time?

    NO   YES

    How frequently?

19. Does your tinnitus change in any way when you

Lie down or bend over	Go up to higher altitude
Sit or stand up quickly	Come down from high altitude
Cough or sneeze	No, None of these actions seems to affect my tinnitus

20. Have you found that any of the following alters your tinnitus?

| Exposure to loud noise | Smoking or other use of tobacco |
| Use of alcohol | Use of marijuana |

Drinking caffeine-containing beverages (coffee, tea, cocoa, cola-type drinks)

No, none of the above alters the tinnitus

21. Does your tinnitus appear to be altered in any way when you

| Are tired | NO | YES | Are relaxed | NO | YES |
| Are tense or nervous | NO | YES | Are in bed at night | NO | YES |

22. Is there anything you know of that changes your tinnitus in any way?

    NO   YES

Attempts to obtain relief

23. Have you prevoiusly sought medical help for your tinnitus?   NO   YES

Indicate briefly where and when

24. Have you previously tried any of the following treatments for tinnitus?

Biofeedback   NO   YES   Give dates

If YES, did you obtain any relief?

Drug Therapy   NO   YES   Give dates

If YES, did you obtain any relief?

Masking   NO   YES   Give dates

If YES, did you obtain any relief?

Hypnosis or acupuncture	NO	YES	Give dates
If YES, did you obtain any relief?			
Any other form of Treatment	NO	YES	Give dates
If YES, did you obtain any relief?			

25. Have you discovered any other form of treatment which seems to help your tinnitus?

For official use only

    Today's date   Examiner

Revised 1-14-83

APPENDIX 4.2

Tinnitus Clinic Questionnaire: History of hearing and ear problems

Name _____ Age _____ Birthdate _____
       Last   First   Initial

26. Have you ever been diagnosed as having any of the following?   NO

                                                Approx Age

    Meniere's disease

    Otosclerosis

    Facial pain, numbness or paralysis

    Cholesteatoma

    Labyrinthitis

    Mastoiditis

27. Have you had any other ear problems or injury   NO   YES

    If yes, please describe, giving dates when possible

28. Do you ever experience the following? (If yes, indicate how often and for how long)

    Dizziness   NO   YES
    Pain in the ear   NO   YES
    Fullness in the ear   NO   YES

29. Do you notice any trouble hearing speech or other types of sound?

    NO   NOT SURE   YES

    If yes, what type of difficulty are you having?

    When did you being to notice difficulty?

    Was the onset of the hearing problem gradual or sudden?

        GRADUAL   SUDDEN
                                          Date of onset—if known

    If it was sudden, was it associated with any of the following?

        Gunfire   Vascular problem

        Explosion   Illness

        Loud music or other loud noise   Other

        Unknown

30. Does your hearing seem to fluctuate?   NO   YES
                                                                       Explain

31. Have you noticed any other changes in how you hear sounds?   NO   YES

                                        Explain

32. Do you find loud sounds more unpleasant than you used to?   NO   YES

    If yes, describe the situations that cause you the most problems

33. Have any of your relatives had problems with their ears or hearing?

    NO   YES Their relationship to you

           What type of problem?

34. Have you ever worn a hearing aid?   NO   YES

                                            Indicate when and for how long

  Worn in   Left ear   Right ear   Both ears

  Make and model (if known)

  How helpful was the hearing amplification?

  Did the hearing aid affect your tinnitus in any way?

35. Which is more of a problem for you, hearing difficulty or tinnitus?

    Hearing difficulty

    Tinnitus

    They're equally bothersome

    Not sure

36. Have you been exposed to loud sounds during any of the following?

    Military service

    Work

    Recreational activities

    Other

37. What is your work?

    How long have you been doing this type of work?

For official use only

Today's date   Examiner

Revised 1-14-83

APPENDIX 4.3

Tinnitus Clinic Questionaire: Medical and Health Information

Name _____   Birthdate _____
     Last   First   Initial   Month   Date   Year

Birthplace _____   Eye color _____   Sex M   F   Righthanded/Lefthanded
                                          (Circle one)   (Circle one)

38. Have you had any of the following?   NO   YES   (check all that apply)

                            Age at onset   Age at onset

    Arthritis or rheumatism   Kidney disease

    High blood pressure   Thyroid problem

    Heart disease   Diabetes

    Blood vessel problem   Hypoglycemia
      (hardening of arteries,
      varicose veins, phlebitis)   Epilepsy (seizures,
                                                                convulsions or other)
    Blood disease

                                                               Stroke
    Lung disease or other
      respiratory problems   Depression

    Other significant medical problem(s) now or in the past
                                                                                         Describe

39a. Please list medications you are currently taking

    Medication name   Amount taken   Frequency   When began taking

39b. When your tinnitus began were you taking any medications?   NO   NOT SURE   YES

    If yes, please list

39c. Have you ever taken an anti-malaria drug such as quinine?   NO   NOT SURE   YES

40. How often do you get headaches?

41a. Have you had any of the following?   NO   YES   (Check all that apply)

                              Approx age   Approx age

    German measles   Chicken pox
      (3-day, rubella)
                                                                Herpes (any form)
    Hard measles
                                                                Mononucleosis
    Mumps
                                                               Hepatitis
    Scarlet fever
                                                               Tuberculosis
    Whooping cough
                                                               Syphilis
    Diptheria
                                                               Malaria
    Rheumatic fever

    Other communicable diseases

ASSESSMENT   95

41b. Apart from the illnesses above, have you even had a severe fever?

    NO   NOT SURE   YES

If yes, please give approximate age

42. Have you ever had a significant head or neck injury   NO   YES

    If yes, please describe and give approximate date(s)

43a. Have you had surgery involving anaesthesia?   NO   YES   NOT SURE

    If yes, please describe and give approximate date(s)

43b. Were you ever hospitalized for any other reason?

                            Please describe and give approximate dates

44. Are you allergic to any of the following?   (If yes, please provide more detail)

    Food   Pollen

    Animal   Drugs

    Other allergies

45. Have you ever had any problems with your teeth or jaw?   NO   YES

    Check all that apply   Jaw pain   Teeth pulled

                                Jaw surgery   Oral surgery

    Do you grind your teeth?   NO   YES

    Do you wear dentures?   NO   YES

    Any other problems with teeth or jaw?

                                                                  Describe briefly

46. Do you smoke or use tobacco in any form?   NO   YES

    Type of tobacco   How often/How much

47. Do you drink alcoholic beverages?   NO   YES

                                                                           How often—how much

48. Do you drink caffeine-containing beverages (coffee, tea, cocoa, cola-type drinks)?

        No   Less than 3 per day   3-6 per day   More than 6 per day

49. Have any of your relatives had the following?   NO   NOT SURE

    Dizziness or vertigo

    Ménière's disease

    Labyrinthitis

    Otosclerosis

    Migraine

    Epilepsy, seizures or fits

    Multiple sclerosis

    Facial pain or numbness

    Other neurological problems

For official use only

5

J. W. P. Hazell

Tinnitus masking therapy

'Why is it that buzzing in the ears ceases if one makes a sound? Is it because a greater sound drives out the less?' This quotation, originally ascribed to Aristotle, is now thought to come from the School of Salerno in the 12th to 13th centuries (Forster 1927). The concept that tinnitus can be helped by the presence of another sound is not new. Itard in 1821 described a number of environmental noises which might be used to help mask tinnitus such as the continuous sound of running water. A clockwork motor placed by the bed and the sound created by damp wood being placed on an open fire. Wilson in 1893 used sounds produced by the newly developed telephone coil to induce residual inhibition and three of his four patients claimed relief although repeated periods of stimulation were required. Jones & Knudsen (1928) described the first electrical tinnitus masker, which took the form of a fairly simple harmonic generator and again only offered temporary relief from tinnitus (see page 17). They noted the ability of tinnitus sufferers to adapt more easily to an external sound than to that of the tinnitus itself. Saltzman & Ersner (1947) discussed the benefit to tinnitus sufferers from hearing-aid fitting, albeit with fairly early instruments, and established that, particularly for those with hearing losses as well, amplified environmental noise could provide a very useful masking effect. However it was not until the pioneering work of Vernon (1977) and his colleagues that a wearable masking device became commercially available. Further details of the history and development of masking therapy may be found in Chapter 1.

THE MECHANISM OF ACOUSTICAL TINNITUS SUPPRESSION

The evidence for a process of active mechanical resonance within the cochlea continues to grow. The subject is addressed in detail in Chapter 2 and is based on the findings of otoacoustic emissions (OAEs) (Kemp 1978). Spontaneous otoacoustic emissions (SOAEs) have also been described by Wilson (1980). The presence of contractile proteins, notably actin and myocin, within the hairs, cuticular plates and supporting cells have been described by Flock and others (1982). Johnstone (1983) considers that the neural and basilar membrane tuning of the cochlea are indeed identical and implies that the inner hair cells are passive and untuned receptors of basilar membrane motion while the outer hair cells provide an active mechanism to sharpen up the basilar membrane response. It is very tempting to think of this source of energy within the cochlea being responsible for some tinnitus, particularly the less complex forms of tonal and broad-band tinnitus.

Wilson (1980) argues in Chapter 2 that there is little clinical correlation between SOAEs and troublesome tinnitus. Nevertheless a useful hypothesis for the generation of some tonal and narrow band tinnitus can be based on this model. In clinical practice the measured pitch of tonal tinnitus is often close to an area of high-frequency hearing loss (Fig. 5.1). This relationship has been pointed out previously by Douek & Reid (1968) who suggested that the tinnitus might be masking the hearing threshold. In Figure 5.1 the high-frequency hearing loss is due to degeneration of hair cells in the basal turn of the cochlea. The outer hair cells in this area are particularly vulnerable to damage by noise or ototoxic drugs. Their demise is the principal cause of high-frequency hearing loss which occurs as a result of the ageing process. The active mechanism argued in Chapter 2 is a device for amplification and frequency detection in the cochlea, particularly at low sound intensities. One might imagine that in a

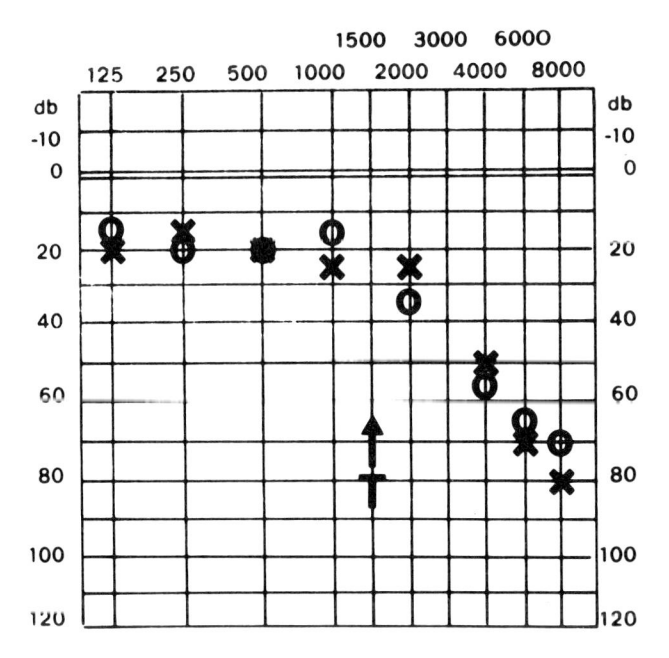

Fig. 5.1 A typical audiogram in sensorineural tinnitus. The arrow (T) indicates the frequency of the tinnitus.

situation where an area of the cochlea has lost this energy, adjacent healthy hair cells, directed by the efferent innervation in the olivo-cochlear bundle, would increase their mechanical (or electromechanical) contribution in an attempt to restore normal function to the basilar membrane. With the exception of SOAEs the normal cochlea is silent, and this mechanical activity is not heard. However such 'compensatory' outer hair cell activity might result in this threshold being exceeded and cochlear tinnitus being created. The common experience of tinnitus being masked by environmental noise could indicate the contribution that such sound energy might make to the stricken area of the basilar membrane. The role of outer hair cells, therefore, is to establish the sharper portion of the cochlear nerve fibre tuning curve rather than the broader response to louder stimuli above 50 dB SPL (sound pressure level), which is mediated more through the mechanical properties of the basilar membrane. Therapeutic tinnitus masking involves the application to the ear of a constant source of white or band-pass noise. This energy could in part exert its suppressing effect by restoring motion to the hair-cell depleted area of the basilar membrane, thus reducing the hyperactivity of outer hair cells in the adjacent part.

The efferent system controlling the outer hair-cell activity is part of the autonomic nervous system (Mendel 1980). It is not difficult to imagine that changes in internal and external stress and variations in circulating adrenalin and vagal tone may have a direct or indirect effect on outer hair-cell activity. In clinical practice tinnitus is often related to stress, anxiety and panic states.

The central auditory pathways undoubtedly have mechanisms similar to those of an electronic automatic gain control. These will tend to increase the sensitivity of the periphery in a quiet environment, increasing outer hair cell activity and tinnitus. This could explain the phenomenon of increased intensity of tinnitus immediately on waking.

After therapeutic masking approximately 10% of patients experience a period of total absence of their tinnitus (total residual inhibition). It is difficult to explain this phenomenon, but if the response of the central auditory mechanism were to be based on a fairly long time constant it is possible that masking might be followed by a period of reduced efferent tone. Although contralateral masking can sometimes be beneficial (and this effect may well be mediated at a cortical level) the acute experiment often results in an increase of tinnitus in the opposite ear. This effect is most probably mediated through the efferent pathways.

This hypothesis is only satisfactory for patients with good residual hearing, at least at some frequencies. Where the cochlea is completely destroyed the hypothesis of Møller (1984) is more attractive. He suggests that a normal silent ear presents a pattern of random neural discharge to the central auditory mechanism. The signals are random in time and with respect to those travelling along adjacent auditory nerve fibres. Loss of myelin insulation on these fibres might result in cross-talk and synchronisation of firing in the nerve which would be heard as tinnitus. A stump neuroma following acoustic nerve section could be expected to have exactly this effect.

These models undoubtedly have many imperfections; however, they have been found very helpful in explaining to the patient why masking therapy might work and in persuading him to take the concept seriously.

INSTRUMENTATION

The prosthetic management of tinnitus involves the selection of one or more of the following instruments:

1. a tinnitus masker;
2. a combination hearing aid and masker (USA: tinnitus instrument);
3. conventional hearing aid.

Tinnitus maskers are devices very similar in appearance to hearing aids (Fig. 5.2) which are worn for the most part post-aurally or all-in-the-ear. More recently, programmable masking devices have become available which involve a larger body-worn device (Figs 5.8, 5.9). The simpler post-aural models incorporate a noise generator (in place of the microphone which would be found in a hearing aid), filters of varying types, an amplifier and transducer. Although attempts have been made to tailor the sound carefully to meet the requirements of those prescribing masking devices, in practice most devices produce a fairly broad band of white noise albeit with a high-frequency emphasis. The problem of measuring the output from maskers has been emphasised by Nunley & Staab (1979) and Martin 1980 (see Hazell & Wood 1981). The apparent frequency response can be varied considerably, depending on the methods of sampling (Figs 5.3-5.5) and also depending on the tone setting (Hazell et al 1985, p. 118). We gained quite a lot of experience in this multicentre trial in which 472 patients were followed through a three-year period with masking instruments of various kinds. On the whole we were pleasantly surprised with the consistency of

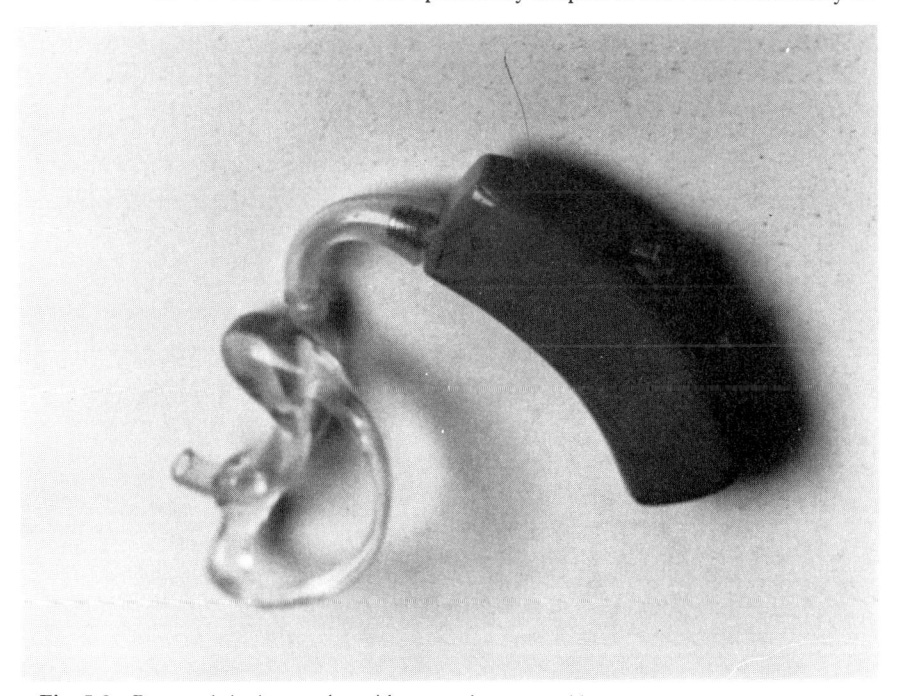

Fig. 5.2 Post-aural tinnitus masker with personal open mould

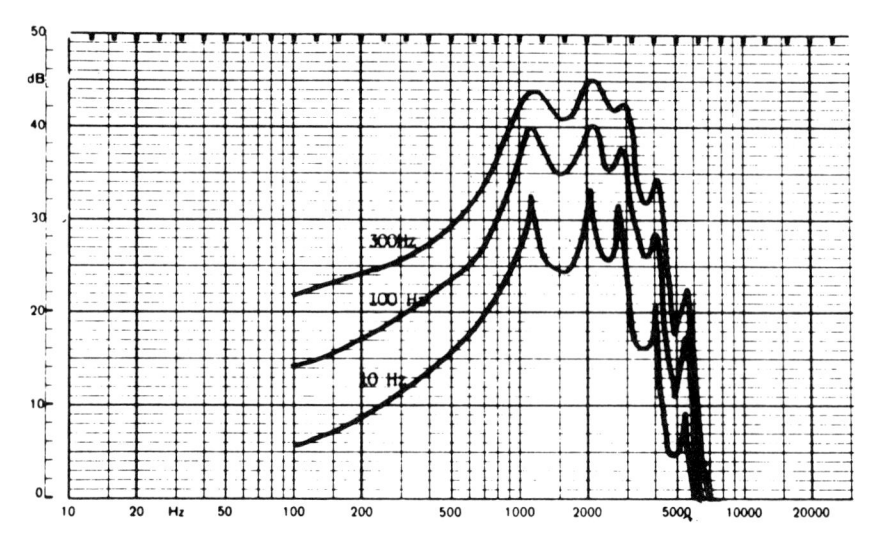

Fig. 5.3 Output from masker analysed with 300, 100 and 10 Hz filter band-widths (from Martin 1980)

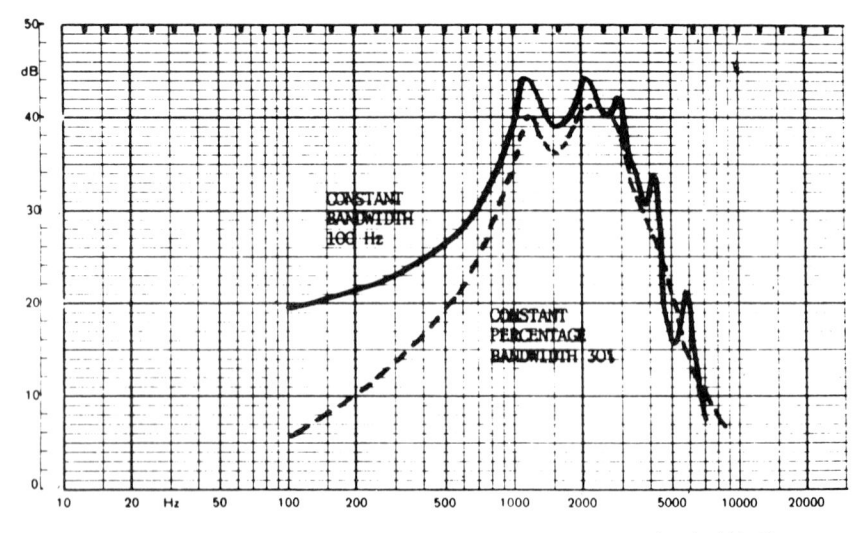

Fig. 5.4 Output from same masker measured with a constant percentage band-width filter (30%) and a constant band-width filter (100 Hz) (from Martin 1980)

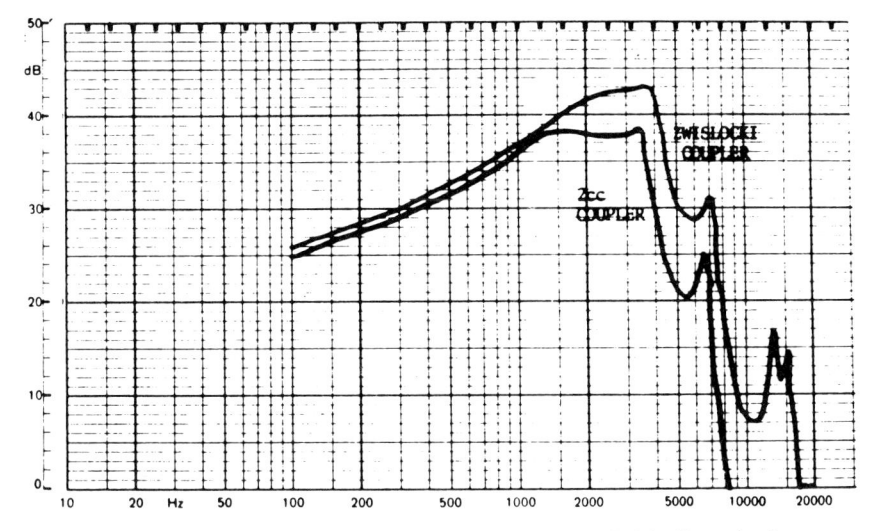

Fig. 5.5 Output from one earphone measured on 2cc coupler and Zwislocki coupler for same input (from Martin 1980)

these instruments and Figure 5.6 shows the output from 75 selected at random (Hazell et al 1985). During the three-year period the maskers proved quite reliable, the worst case being an incidence of 6% of major repairs required against 11% for the hearing aids used. The combination hearing aid and masker unit which we used had two separate parts (Fig. 5.7) which made it less reliable (14% required major repairs).

It is essential that patients fitted with maskers should rapidly adapt to the sound that the masker makes. If the noise is 'smooth' and constant this process of adaptation is much faster than if there tend to be fluctuations in the output, or a 'rough' sound resulting from a less than random noise generator.

SELECTION OF PATIENTS

No-one would deny that tinnitus as a symptom is a common cause of referral to otologists, audiologists, neurologists and other physicians. The high incidence of this complaint has been identified by the MRC Insitute of Hearing Research (Ch. 3). In the multicentre study of tinnitus masking (Hazell et al 1985) a total of 668 patients were seen initially, of whom 472 were deemed suitable for entry into the study over a three-year period: 8% were rejected because tinnitus was clearly not a major problem and no further management was required besides reassurance in a clinic setting. In a study by Schleuning et al (1980) 102 out of a total of 578 patients with tinnitus were not recommended masking treatment, but this included some patients who had been given an acute test with a masker to determine their suitability. The proportion of

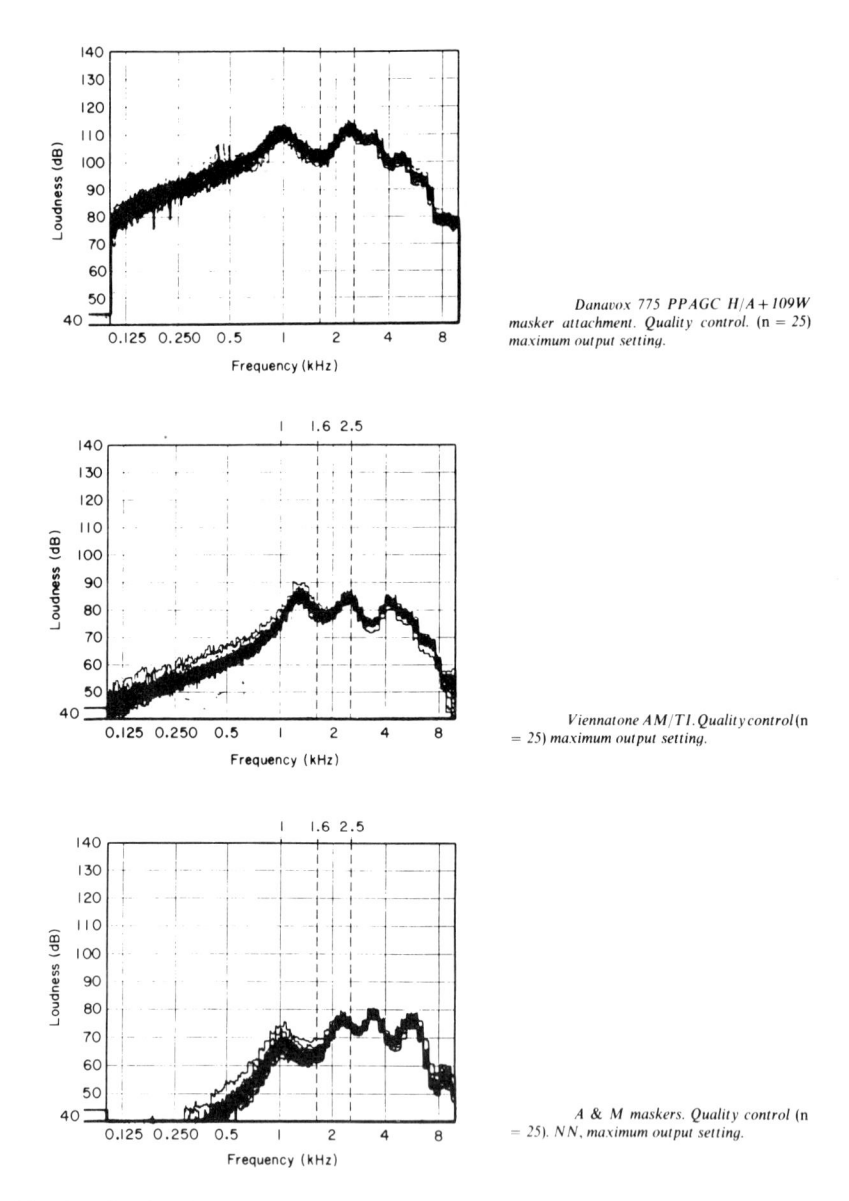

Fig. 5.6 Bruel & Kjaer audio test centre types 2624, ½" microphone and test station type 2116. Standard 2 cc coupler (from Hazell et al 1985)

Danavox 775 PPAGC H/A+109W masker attachment. Quality control. (n = 25) maximum output setting.

Viennatone AM/TI. Quality control (n = 25) maximum output setting.

A & M maskers. Quality control (n = 25). NN, maximum output setting.

patients recommended for masking therapy will depend on the facilities available, e.g. the availability of masking instruments and suitably trained therapists. Nevertheless the large majority of patients having sensorineural tinnitus as their major complaint should be considered for a masking programme and many of these will undoubtedly obtain benefit (Hazell et al 1985, Vernon & Schleuning 1978, McFadden 1982).

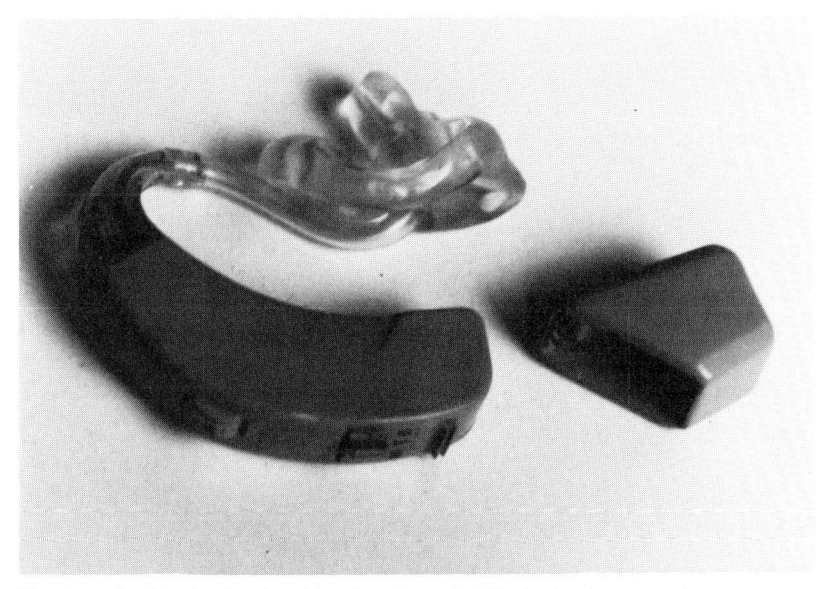

Fig. 5.7 Combination hearing aid and masker unit (US: tinnitus instrument)

Clinical selection criteria

A tinnitus clinic was established at University College Hospital, London in 1977. By 1985 about 2000 patients had been seen, of whom two-thirds have received fittings of masking instruments. Our clinic is organized so that the patients are seen jointly by the otologist and tinnitus therapist, in our case an audiological scientist. Decisions about the initial therapeutic approach are discussed between doctor and therapist at the end of the consultation, together with alternatives that might be tried if this is unsuccessful. The therapist is introduced to the patient at this early stage and a full explanation is given of the mechanism of the tinnitus generation, as far as this is known, and the treatment or therapy which is considered to be most appropriate.

History taking is a most important part, perhaps *the* most important part, of the patient's assessment, as symptomatic treatment can only be effective if it alleviates patients' distress. In the past it has been the experience of many tinnitus sufferers that little attention is paid to the presenting symptom. It is important to encourage the patient to talk about tinnitus and how it affects his life and work. Most patients are anxious and a relaxed environment, together with the provision of any communication aids that may be necessary if they have a hearing loss, will help them to talk. The temporal factors of the patient's tinnitus, such as its overall duration, remissions and fluctuations, cannot be measured audiometrically, and detailed notes should be made of these points as they may well affect the way in which any programme of masking therapy is applied. It is important to elicit the nature and number of different sounds and their locations, particularly identifying which is the most troublesome tinnitus. Often multiple sounds exist, many of which have been present for some years and do not cause distress. The apparent loudness of the tinnitus and in particular the effect of environmental masking noise may well act as a guide to the help that therapeutic masking will give.

It is important to assess the effect of tinnitus on the patient's activities, particularly whether concentration is impaired or whether mental activity is sufficient to distract from the presence of the tinnitus. Many patients who are unaware of their tinnitus during the day may be severely affected in the evening when they might otherwise be looking forward to a period of quiet recreational activity. The inability to enjoy this period of relaxation with their family or friends can very much reduce the quality of life. The majority of our patients use their maskers for this period only. Sleep disturbance is a big problem among tinnitus patients although it is not a measure of the severity of the tinnitus itself (Institute of Hearing Research 1981); often patients slept badly prior to the onset of tinnitus. For those whose tinnitus makes getting off to sleep difficult, or who cannot get back to sleep on waking in the night, a period of masking can be very helpful in inducing the relaxation necessary for normal sleep. Many patients are profoundly depressed and as a result may wake early in the morning, a time when the environment is very quiet and their tinnitus most prominent.

It is most important to assess the patient's communication abilities. Although 27% of our patients have hearing within normal limits for their age (Hazell et al 1985, see also Heller & Bergmann 1953) two-thirds of patients with hearing impairment are troubled by tinnitus (Office of Population Censuses and Surveys 1983). It is a common experience that patients with a primary hearing loss and communication difficulty will stress their tinnitus as a cause of the problem: 'Tinnitus is worse when I am in a crowd of people and I can't hear what's being said'. It may be very hard to persuade patients that the tinnitus is related to the hearing loss and not the other way round. Nevertheless tinnitus may interfere with concentration, and cause anxiety, which makes communication more difficult. It is obviously important to unravel which problem – the tinnitus or the hearing loss – is the major complaint, and decide whether tinnitus therapy or hearing rehabilitation is the most appropriate first line of action.

Audiometric investigations

The point has been frequently made that the only means of telling which patients are going to benefit from therapeutic masking is to institute a clinical trial in each case (Hazell & Wood 1981, Vernon & Meikle 1981, Sheldrake et al 1985). Hazell et al (1985) looked in detail at the predictive value of various audiological measurements of tinnitus. A comparison was made between these criteria and the answers to the question asked of each patient at the end of the study: 'Whilst wearing the instrument, did it help to mask the tinnitus?'. Answers were according to a 5-point scale: 1=all the time, 2=three-quarters of the time, 3=half the time, 4=one quarter of the time, 5=never. The results are shown in Table 5.1. There was a just significant relationship between the ability of white noise to mask the tinnitus ear in an acute experiment and the effectiveness of a tinnitus masker applied therapeutically. This significance was also seen at the $p=0.05$ level when this measurement of masking was

Table 5.1 Tinnitus measurements as a predictor of therapeutic masking success (from Hazell et al 1985)

	Correlation coefficient	n	Significance
TEPTA	0.09	203	
TEWBNT	0.04	116	
TEWBNIM	0.09	181	
TEWBNML	0.15	187	$p = 0.05$
TEWBNMSL	0.04	184	
TEMLDIFF	0.07	173	
TEULL	0.03	195	
TEMLDR	0.19	108	$p = 0.05$
TEIMDR	−0.10	110	

TEPTA Average pure tone audiometric threshold; TEWPNT Wide-band noise threshold; TEWBIM Wide-band noise intensity match; TEWBNML Wide-band noise minimal masking level (dB HL); TEWBNMSL Wide-band noise minimal masking level (dB sensation level); TEMLDIFF Difference between tinnitus intensity match and minimal masking level; TEULL Uncomfortable loudness level of white noise; TEMLDR Wide-band noise minimal masking level expressed as a percentage of the dynamic range of the ear; TEIMDR Tinnitus intensity match expressed as a percentage of the dynamic range of the ear. All measurements performed in the ear with the more troublesome tinnitus.

expressed as a percentage of dynamic range of the ear. Although these measurements are probably useful in determining the masking effects of white noise in an individual from time to time, or in comparing the effects of masking on one ear or the other, the correlation coefficients are very low for such a large study and if these tests are used as predictors of which patients will benefit from masking therapy or not, then many patients who might be helped will be sent away.

The initial work of Vernon and others (Vernon 1977) suggested that the major advantage of masking was that periods of total relief from tinnitus occurred on removing the masking instrument. The term 'residual inhibition' (Feldmann 1971) has been used to describe this effect. A test was devised by Vernon (see Ch. 4) using MML +10 dB for 60 seconds. Hazell et al (1985) employed this in their study, and show a relationship between the acute test and the experience of residual inhibition after therapeutic masking, but only in relation to complete or total inhibition. The effect of a partial reduction of the tinnitus level after masking is also beneficial to the patients and occurs more frequently. Total residual inhibition occurred only in 10% of our patients (Table 5.2). Neither Vernon nor Hazell now recommend that patients should be counselled on the basis of the likelihood that a broad-band masker will produce residual inhibition. However the spectrum of

Table 5.2. Result of residual inhibition (RI) test against R.I. experience after therapeutic masking (from Hazell et al 1985)

	R.I. experience after therapeutic masking (%)				
Result of R.I. test	Tinnitus disappeared	Tinnitus quieter	Tinnitus unchanged	Tinnitus louder	No. of subjects
Tinnitus completely gone	25	22	47	6	32
Loudness reduced	9	36	43	13	56
No change	5	31	60	4	88
Loudness enhanced	0	42	50	8	12

masking required to provide continuous relief while the instrument is being worn ('continuous masking') is likely to be different to the spectrum which will produce optimal residual inhibition. Terry et al (1983) in acute experiments showed that residual inhibition depended on the central frequency of the masker which was usually lower than the tinnitus frequency. It also varied between subjects, and was proportional to the masker intensity provided that the tinnitus was completely masked. Residual inhibition could not be produced by contralateral masking. They suggested that when residual inhibition occurred it was accompanied by a temporary threshold shift around the tinnitus frequency. Hazell et al (1985) confirmed the previous finding of Vernon that hearing aids never produced total residual inhibition. It was also worth noting that in this study hearing aids made tinnitus louder after their removal in 24% of cases, as opposed to 7% among the wearers of tinnitus maskers. Harris and Mollestrom (1984) have determined that the most effective stimulus for producing residual inhibition therapeutically is one which most closely simulates the tinnitus itself. To this purpose they have developed a programmable masker (Figs. 5.8, 5.9) and a strategy of using these masking sounds for short periods during the day to induce residual inhibition (Mollestrom et al 1984).

Hazell & Wood (1981) suggest that a broad-band signal is more appropriate for effective continuous masking. Comparisons of appropriate masking signals as may be determined by Feldmann masking curves, with the central frequency of the tinnitus itself, show poor correlation (Fig. 5.10). Feldmann (1971) himself suggests that white noise is a more effective masker in the acute experiment than pure tones or narrow bands for the majority of cases. It is therefore important to decide what strategy is being followed, depending on whether the desired effect is primarily one of

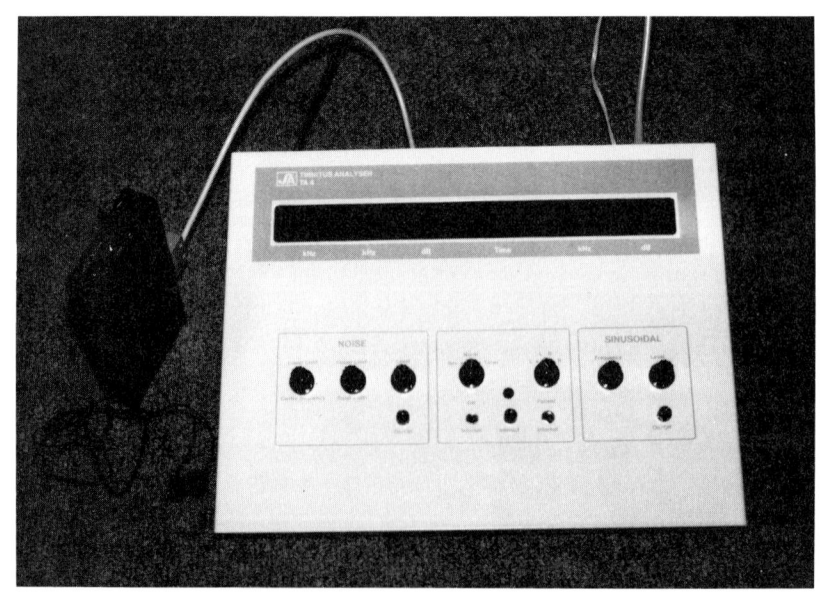

Fig. 5.8 Programmable masker by Scandinavia Audiometer AB, Box 16015, S-200 25 Malmö, Sweden

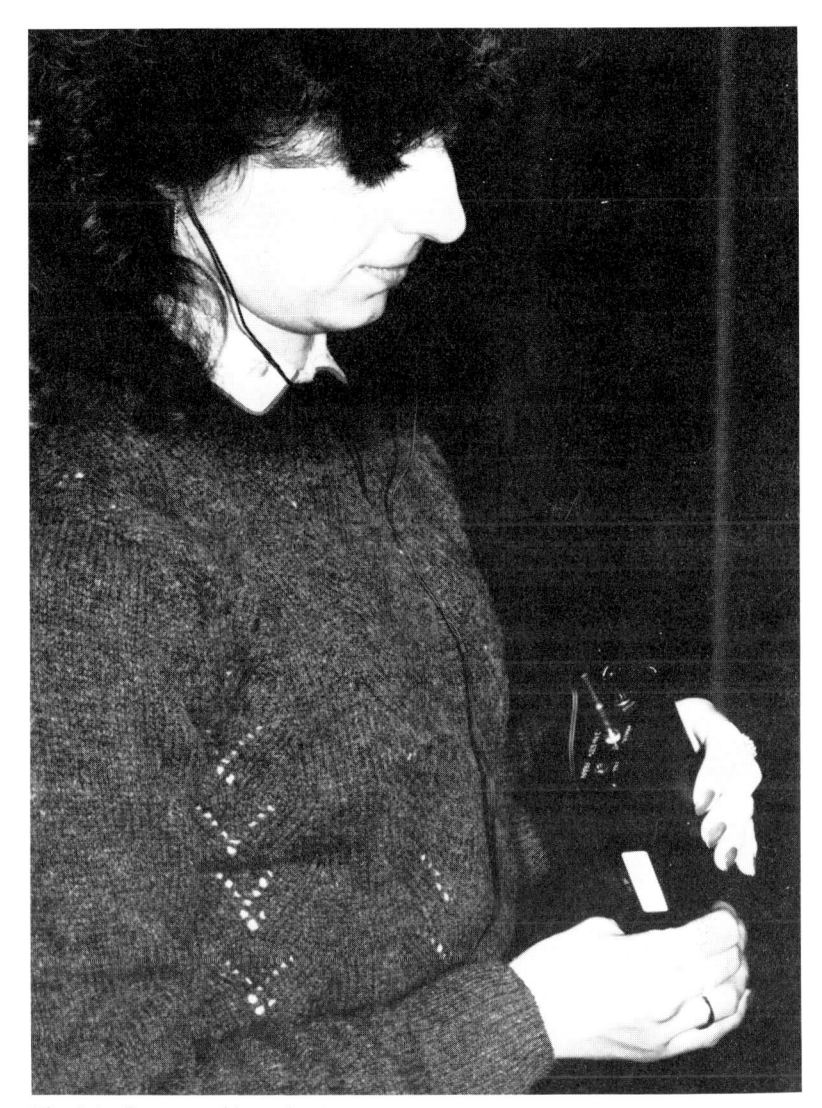

Fig. 5.9 Programmable masker in use

continuous masking, or one of residual inhibition. We have not found the measurement of the tinnitus frequency any help in determining the effectiveness of continuous masking or in indicating what the spectrum of such masking should be (Hazell et al 1985). The most appropriate audiometric investigation is likely to be one in which the effects of different masking sounds on the tinnitus are observed. Even so, there are patients who benefit from masking simply from the provision of another distracting background sound, and in whom the masking sound does not completely cover the tinnitus. The counsel of perfection is to provide a therapeutic trial of masking for all patients.

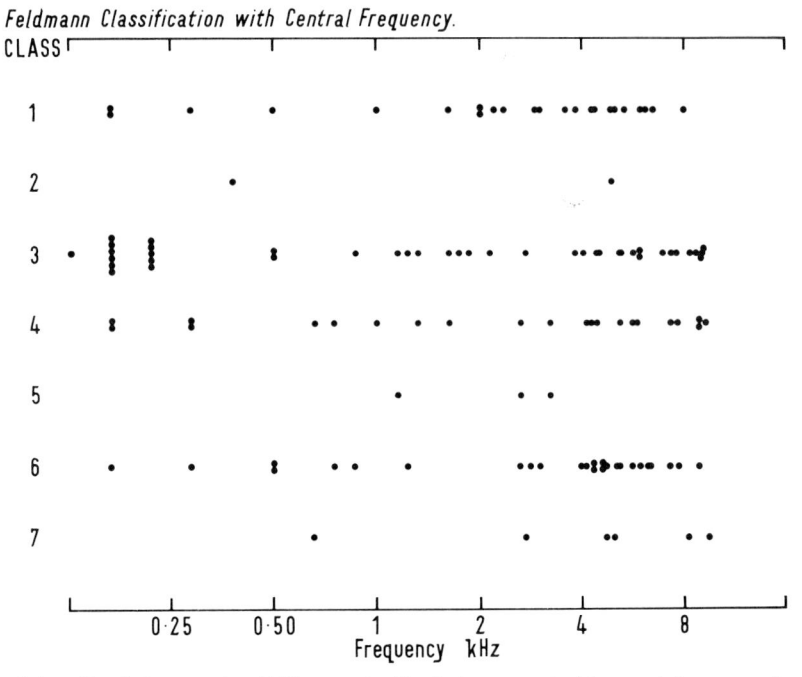

Fig. 5.10 Signals from masker (Feldmann classification) compared with central frequency of tinnitus (from Hazell 1985)

The influence of other pathologies

The importance of proper investigation and diagnosis is emphasised by Vernon and by Goodey in Chapters 4 and 10 and every effort should be made to establish the predisposing cause for the development of tinnitus in an individual. This is important not only to satisfy the patient's natural desire for an explanation, but also because treatment of relevant co-existing systemic conditions may influence the tinnitus itself.

An important part of our diagnostic activities in the tinnitus clinic involves the exclusion of arteriopathy, thyroid dysfunction, anaemia, deficiencies of zinc and vitamin B, syphilis and acoustic neuroma. Objective measurements are made with a stethoscope (Tewfik 1984) and an intra-meatal microphone (Hazell 1984). In practice, however, other systemic disease is established in less than 20% of our tinnitus population and its effective treatment does not necessarily mean an improvement in the tinnitus. The tinnitus of cochlear otosclerosis, particularly where it seems likely that the source of sound is a vascular one in an otosclerotic focus, may respond to sodium fluoride treatment and this is certainly worth trying for a six-month period (Causse et al 1981, Shambaugh 1977). The tinnitus of Ménière's disease may well remit with improvement in low-frequency hearing as a result of medical or surgical treatment. In the initial stages of the disease the tinnitus is often less troublesome than the vertigo or hearing loss, but in advanced cases where there is a considerable hearing loss the tinnitus may be very troublesome. Vernon, Johnson & Schleuning 1981 and Hazell and Wood (1981) have reported the relative ease with which the tinnitus of Ménière's disease may be masked. In Ménière's disease it is worth trying masking strategies, even in the presence of a profound hearing loss.

Recruitment and Hyperacusis

Many patients with tinnitus also have severe loudness discomfort, and our initial reaction was that they were unlikely to be helped by masking therapy. In the event nothing proved further from the truth, indeed it was possible to demonstrate a great reduction of loudness discomfort in those patients with recruitment who used maskers on a continuous basis. It seemed that the gradual and continuous introduction of sound into the ear to some extent desensitised it to the effects of loud sound. Many patients wear ear muffs and plugs continuously in an attempt to avoid the unpleasant effects of sound and the subsequent increase of their tinnitus. It cannot be overstressed how counterproductive these measures are. The ear becomes increasingly more sensitive, so that any sound in the environment becomes unbearable, and patients become progressively more and more isolated. Some patients have loudness discomfort levels at between 40 and 50 dB HL (hearing level) to pure tones. A programme of masking should be instituted which begins with low levels of masking sound applied at quiet times for two to three hours a day, increasing the levels of masking and its duration, and monitoring carefully the loudness discomfort levels on audiometry. We are now using this technique for patients with and without tinnitus, who have severe loudness recruitment (Hazell & Sheldrake 1986). Some of these patients have fairly normal hearing, but others with hearing losses are helped by this technique to make better use of amplification.

MASKER FITTING

After the first consultation at the tinnitus clinic a decision is made between otologist and therapist as to whether or not the patient is suitable for tinnitus masking. We believe there is a great advantage to be gained in arranging for the masker fittings and patient counselling to take place under the auspices of the clinic where the patient first receives otological guidance. However the practice will vary, particularly in the United States where patients may be referred for this to a hearing aid practitioner (Schleuning et al 1980). At the first visit we take ear mould impressions from both ears of the patient in most cases. This makes it possible to start immediately with the therapeutic trial at the next visit, and allows for a change in strategy either to contralateral or binaural masking at any time.

Choice of ear mould

Over 95% of our patients are fitted with open moulds (Hazell & Wood 1981) which leave the ear canal as far as possible completely unoccluded. A light skeleton mould design is preferred as many patients with tinnitus dislike having the feeling of anything in the affected ear. A solid or inadequately vented mould will produce an ear plug effect even before the masking device is switched on tending to make the tinnitus louder. Fitting of a masker with an occluding mould is the most common single cause of failure in masking therapy that we have encountered. The effect of fitting the masker with an open mould also enhances the high-frequency component, which helps to produce better continuous masking, and is less likely to interfere with hearing (at least in quiet situations) (Spitzer et al 1983) as most of the energy will be above the speech frequency spectrum. The tubing should be left long, initially, in the intrameatal part, as this can be used to help alter the frequency spectrum and intensity of masking sound. If fairly high levels of masking noise are required to achieve a therapeutic effect, too short a tube may result in the masker being heard by others with subsequent embarrassment to the patient. With profound hearing losses or very severe tinnitus an occlusive mould may be needed, although a vent should always be employed wherever possible. It should be remembered that the sound pressure level delivered to the ear will rise dramatically if this is done, and if in addition high-powered maskers are used great care should be taken that this does not result in any threshold shift in the hearing. Such fitting should be under the direction of a physician only, and frequent serial audiometry performed during the follow-up period.

STRATEGY FOR MASKER FITTING

The strategy currently employed in our tinnitus clinic is summarised in the flow diagram (Fig. 5.11). Hazell et al (1985) have stressed the importance of correcting any significant hearing loss. In practice, and particularly with older patients, this often involves the fitting of binaural, post-aural high-frequency hearing aids with open moulds. However, tinnitus suppression with hearing aids is generally less effective than with maskers and in any case patients may require tinnitus suppression most at times when there is no environmental sound to amplify. In many cases this requires the fitting first of all of suitable hearing aids to improve hearing, and also the fitting of a masking device for use in the evening or at night time when all is quiet. The decision about which to do first will require a careful assessment of which symptom is really most troublesome to the patient. A surprising number of patients end up wearing a masker in one ear and a hearing aid in the other. This may give better tinnitus suppression than two maskers in some bilateral cases, as well as improving hearing.

In cases of hearing loss where tinnitus relief is not achieved by a hearing aid alone, combination instruments (tinnitus instruments) can be very effective (Fig. 5.7). However they tend to be larger and have more controls, leading to handling difficulties. Fit the instrument as a hearing aid first, before instructing on its use as a masker. All-in-the-ear or canal hearing aids and tinnitus maskers are becoming increasingly popular for cosmetic reasons and ease of handling. Great care must be taken with such fittings to leave the tinnitus ear as widely vented as possible. For this reason canal aids are often found unsuitable.

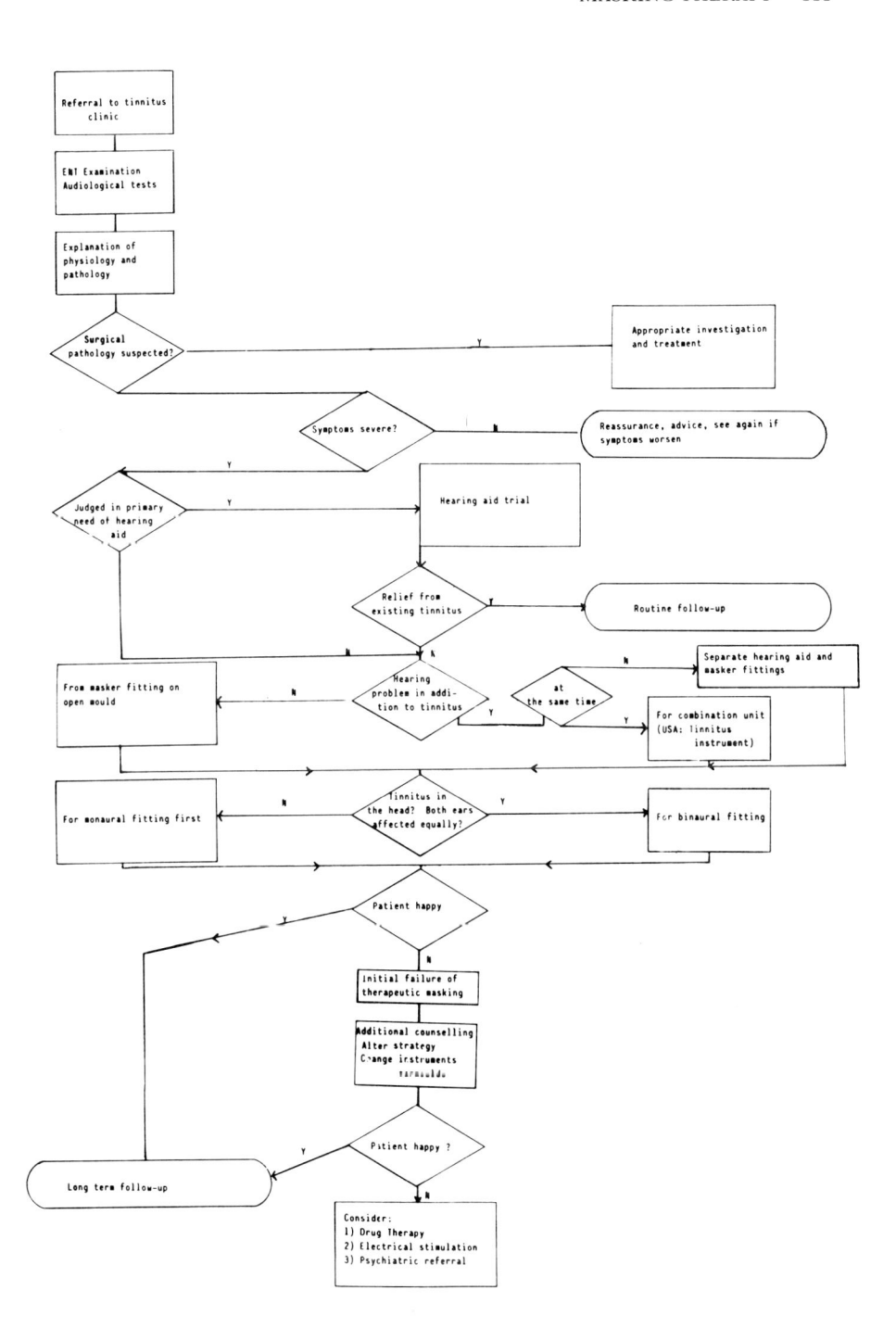

Fig. 5.11 Patient management at the tinnitus clinic at University College Hospital, London

Which ear to mask

In unilateral tinnitus the tinnitus ear is almost invariably the most approrpiate to mask. The exception here will be a dead ear or one with such a profound loss that the masking sound cannot be heard. Contralateral masking is not very effective in our experience and currently we have only six or seven patients using contralateral maskers successfully. Tinnitus in a dead ear accounts for the majority of patients that we are unable to help in any way. In binaural tinnitus it is important to establish whether this is predominantly in one ear, equally in both ears, or heard as a meld of sound within the head. Where the tinnitus is bilateral but asymmetrical we start by masking the most severely affected ear. Sometimes this results in effective symptom control, and at other times the tinnitus in the untreated ear becomes the predominant symptom. It is difficult to know whether in these cases masking actually increases the level of tinnitus in the contralateral ear or whether with the control of tinnitus in one ear that in the other becomes more noticeable. In such cases subsequent fitting of a second masker to the other ear must be tried. In symmetrical tinnitus and tinnitus heard within the head it is best to tell the patient that binaural masking is essential for symptom control.

The question of whether to attempt a binaural fitting at the initial therapy session or to leave the second fitting to a subsequent appointment has not been resolved (Sheldrake et al 1985). Fitting a single instrument does run the risk of leaving the patient with uncontrolled tinnitus in the other ear, and the patient must be carefully counselled that this may occur. It does, however, get over the problems of learning to use two instruments at once and many older patients in this situation have real handling difficulties. In the UCH tinnitus clinic both strategies have been used at different times with successful results.

Introducing the patient to the masker

The patient needs to become familiar with the way in which the masker works – the volume control, battery compartment, connections to ear mould etc. – and be shown how to introduce the mould successfully into the ear. So far the techniques will be well known to those experienced with hearing-aid fittings.

After placing the instrument in the patient's ear, it is switched on and the volume advanced to the point at which the masking sound is heard by the patient (Masking Sensation Level—MSL). It is then advanced to the point where the patient's tinnitus becomes just inaudible (Minimum Masking Level—MML). A note is made of the points at which the MSL and MML are reached by making a small mark on the volume control or noting the numbered settings. In most cases the patient can be encouraged by the very low level of masking noise that is necessary to cover the tinnitus and make it inaudible. In some cases the tinnitus tends to 'break through' the masking noise and this can lead to the instrument being continually turned up, 'chasing' the tinnitus until the level of masking required becomes intolerable. It is much better to leave the tinnitus masker at its initial setting where the tinnitus is just audible through the masking sound and to initially approach with a strategy of 'a background distracting sound' rather than one which totally masks the patient's tinnitus. This criteria for tinnitus relief, although not as dramatic as completely masking the tinnitus, is nevertheless effective for many patients (Hazell et al 1985). Moreover patients will find that there are times when this breakthrough effect does not occur, and that better control may be achieved after a longer period of therapeutic masking.

COUNSELLING

We estimate that over half our patients would never come for help with their tinnitus if it were not for the presence of coexisting stress, anxiety or depressive illness which makes this symptom unbearable. It is fruitless and unrealistic to approach the tinnitus in isolation. It is inevitable that the patients' other fears, worries and anxieties will interreact with the symptom of tinnitus in many different ways, although they may at first lack insight into this. The therapist involved in counselling must decide how far he or she is able to go in attempting to resolve these other problems and conflicts. So often there are business, financial and domestic worries which in analysis prove to be far less bearable than the tinnitus itself. However the otological symptom and subsequent referral may be more acceptable to the patient than presenting with a psychological or psychiatric complaint. For part of the session general counselling techniques may be most helpful. Our tinnitus therapists have benefited in this respect from courses in general counselling, although it must be stressed that many of the techniques used in general counselling are quite useless when it comes to specific counselling about tinnitus itself. In general counselling one approach (Rogers 1961) is to answer a question with another, or turn the question around, so that the patient ends up trying to answer the question himself. This strategy is unhelpful in dealing with specific questions about how tinnitus may be managed. It is often only during counselling sessions that the true extent of other problems becomes apparent, and if these prove to be beyond the capabilities of the therapist the patient should be referred back to the original clinic with a view to cross-referral for more expert psychological or psychiatric help. Despite the frequency of such problems, this course of action is necessary in under 2% of patients receiving masking therapy in our clinic.

Masker counselling

On the first session when the ear mould impression is taken there must be an opportunity for the therapist to outline the patient's masking programme. An idea is needed of the frequency of visits and what these will entail. Already most patients have a number of questions which they forgot to ask during the course of the first consultation and all should be recommended to make written notes which can be brought to these sessions.

Reassurance

Many patients need constant, almost repetitive reassurance that their tinnitus is due to a benign pathology. Many are obsessed with the fear of brain tumour, or of an imminent stroke or psychiatric condition. In turn, discussion about the hypothesis of tinnitus generation may be helpful.

Explanation of masking principles

Where maskers or combination instruments are being fitted there are a number of key points which can be made. The initial attitude may be a rather negative one: that a second masking sound is simply to be added to that of the patient's tinnitus. It is important to stress the ways in which the patient is likely to be helped:

1. The masking sound, although audible, is most often effective at an apparent intensity much less than that of the patient's tinnitus.
2. It is an external noise which is much less obtrusive than the internally generated tinnitus and rapid adaptation to the masking sound is to be expected.
3. It is a steady noise which does not fluctuate either in intensity or frequency as the patient's tinnitus may do.
4. It is a noise without meaning or significance, and is therefore better at masking the tinnitus than a radio or television which may provide a distraction and reduce concentration on another task.
5. The masking sound, unlike the patient's tinnitus, is completely under the individual's control. It may be turned up or down or off at will.
6. It has a generally soothing and calming effect. White noise has been used as an adjunct to the induction of anaesthesia and may have a mild tranquillizing effect.
7. There may be beneficial long-term effects. As the patient focuses less attention on the tinnitus while it is masked, it may become less troublesome and obtrusive when the masker is removed, even in the absence of any inhibition effects. Many of our patients who have had tinnitus for twenty years or more and have never adapted to it appear able to adapt, even at this late stage, after a period of therapeutic masking.
8. Patients should realise that maximum benefit may not be achieved immediately. Some patients only manage to learn to control their tinnitus with masking, and adapt to the masking sound, after two or three months of masker use.
9. Residual inhibition. With our current masking techniques, particularly those employing narrow or broad-band noise, it is unwise to pin too much of the patient's hopes on achieving residual inhibition. However, it is fair to say that just under 10% will have short periods of complete freedom and 30-40% will have periods of reduced tinnitus following masking.
10. Reassurance should be given that masking has not been shown to produce any change in the hearing. Many patients alrady have fears that their tinnitus indicates ensuing deafness, and reassurance should be given that there is no evidence for this (Hazell et al 1985).

PLANNING A PROGRAMME

After the first consultation the initial fitting session will be of paramount importance. We feel at least an hour should be allowed for this as there is usually a great deal of ground to cover and it is important that patients leave with a positive attitude to masking therapy, even if they realise that maximum benefit may not be achieved at once. The importance of keeping follow-up appointments should be stressed even if the patient feels that little improvement is being made. Spouses should be encouraged to attend, learn how the treatment works and participate in the supportive measures.

The first follow-up visit should be arranged at about one month. In the initial stages it is quite helpful for the patient to keep a diary or progress report of how the instrument has helped. This will allow a more objective view of the effectiveness of masking and also identify any special problems that the patient has. Check that the patient has mastered the use of the instrument, and any control adjustments; ear mould modifications or change in types of instrument can be made at this point. Long-term diary keeping is discouraged as this tends to work against the process of adaptation to the tinnitus. Further reassurance about benign pathology, encouragement about the use of the instruments and general supportive measures are nearly always needed at this and subsequent couselling sessions. An adequate time must be alloted to achieve good overall results. Further sessions, which should be of at least half an hour each, will be arranged according to the individual needs of the patient and also logistical requirements; many of our patients travel long distances and are elderly.

Repeat audiometry at least at six-monthly intervals is recommended, particularly in those patients who are using high levels of masking noise. A proportion of patients will have a progressive element to their hearing loss relating to the underlying pathology, and the need for additional auditory rehabilitation must always be borne in mind.

In planning how and when each patient will use their masker or maskers it is essential to have a clear picture of the disability caused in each case. Many patients have no problems at all during the day when tinnitus is masked by environmental noise, and may only need to wear their maskers for relief during quiet recreational periods in the evening, or with help in getting to sleep at night. Other patients with primary sleeping difficulties may be encouraged to wear their maskers immediately before going to sleep, or even keep them on during the night. Sleeping with a masker in is easier for some people than others, and special attention to the fitting, comfort of ear mould, and stability of the instrument behind the ear is needed. An alternative strategy is to have the masker by the bed so that on waking in the night it may be easily inserted to provide immediate relief before tension builds up and further sleep becomes impossible. In those patients in whom tinnitus is constantly troublesome throughout the day, the masker should be introduced slowly for a couple of hours at first and then increased until it is being worn all the time. We have at least twenty patients in follow-up who have been wearing their maskers continuously for a period of over seven years (without significant threshold shift, and with continued and continuous relief).

SUMMARY

With each programme of masking it is important to remember

1. That fitting and counselling strategies for tinnitus must be learnt by experience and contact with tinnitus patients. They cannot be assumed to be adequate as the result of an ability to rehabilitate hearing impairment successfully.
2. That masking therapy cannot be said to have failed until every combination or permutation of masking devices and/or hearing aids has been tried (Fig. 5.11).

Acknowledgement

I am deeply grateful to Pat Garrett for taking this chapter through its many drafts, providing expert help with illustrations and for preparing the manuscript in its final form.

REFERENCES

Causse J R, Uriel J, Berges J, Bretlau P, Causse J B 1981 Mecanisme enzymatique de d'otospongiose. Action du NaF. Annales d'Oto-Laryngologie 98: 269–297

Douek E, Reid J 1968 The diagnostic value of tinnitus pitch. Journal of Laryngology 82: 1039–1042

Feldmann H. 1971 Homolateral and contralateral masking of tinnitus by noise-bands and pure tones. Audiology (Basel) 10: 138–144

Flock A, Bretscher A, Weber K, 1982 Immunohistochemical localisation of several cytoskeletal proteins in inner ear sensory and supporting cells. Hearing Research 7: 75–89

Forster E S 1927 Problemata. In Ross W D (ed) The works of Aristotle. Clarendon, Oxford

Harris S, Mollestrom B 1984 Tinnitus analyzer/masker – clinical experiences. Proceedings of the Tinnitus Seminar, Uppsala Nov 1983. Swedish Council for Planning and Co-ordination of Research, pp 151–160

Hazell J W P 1984 Spontaneous cochlear acoustic emissions and tinnitus: Clinical experience in the tinnitus patient. Journal of Laryngology Supplement 9, pp 106–110.

Hazell J W P 1985 Management of tinnitus: discussion paper. Journal of the Royal Society of Medicine 78: 56–60

Hazell J W P, Sheldrake J B 1986 Unpublished observations

Hazell J W P, Wood S M 1981 Tinnitus masking. A significant contribution to tinnitus management. British Journal of Audiology 15: 223–230

Hazell J W P, Wood S M, Cooper H R et al 1985 A clinical study of tinnitus maskers. British Journal of Audiology 19: 65–146

Heller M F, Bergman M 1953 Tinnitus aurium in normally hearing persons. Annals of Otology 62: 73–83

Itard J M G 1821 Traité des maladies de l'oreille et de l'audition. Mequignon-Marvis, Paris

Johnstone B M 1983 Mechanics of the mammalian cochlea. Proceedings of the International Union of Physiological Sciences (Sydney) 15: 113.01

Institute of Hearing Research 1981 Population study of hearing disorders in adults. Preliminary communication. Journal of the Royal Society of Medicine 74: 819–827

Jones I H, Knudsen V O 1928 Certain aspects of tinnitus, particularly treatment. Laryngoscope 38: 597–611

Kemp D T 1981 Stimulated acoustic emissions from the human auditory system. Journal of the Acoustical Society of America 64: 1386–1391

Kemp D T 1981 Physiologically active cochlear micro-mechanics: one source of tinnitus. In: Evered D, Lawrenson G (eds) Tinnitus. Ciba Foundation Symposium 85. Pitman, London, pp 54–76

Martin M C 1980 Tinnitus maskers. British Tinnitus Association Newsletter No. 6 p 1–6
McFadden D 1982 Tinnitus: facts, theories and treatments. National Academy Press, Washington DC
Mendel D 1980 A basis for the pharmacology of hearing. Journal of Laryngology 94: 1363–1376
Moller A R 1984 Pathophysiology of tinnitus. Annals of Otology Rhinology and Laryngology 93: 39–44
Mollestrom B, Harris S, Andersson M 1984 Tinnitus analyzer/masker–technical presentation and investigation methods. Proceedings of the Tinnitus Seminar, Uppsala Nov 1983. Swedish Council for Planning and Co-ordination of Research, pp 144–150
Nunley J, Staab W J 1979 How to read tinnitus masker data. Hearing Instruments 30(9): 28, 29, 48
Office of Population Censuses and Surveys 1983 General Household survey. The prevalence of tinnitus 1981. GHS 83/1, OPCS, London
Rogers C R 1961 On becoming a person. Houghton Mifflin, Boston
Saltzman M, Ersner M S 1947 A hearing aid for the relief of tinnitus aurium. Laryngoscope 57: 358–366
Schleuning A J, Johnson R M, Vernon J A 1980 Evaluation of a tinnitus masking program: a follow-up study of 598 patients. Ear and Hearing 1: 71–74
Shambaugh G E Jr 1977 Further experiences with moderate dosage of sodium fluoride for sensorineural hearing loss, tinnitus and vertigo due to otospongiosis. Advances in Oto-Rhino-Laryngology 22: 35–42
Sheldrake J B, Wood S M, Cooper H R 1985 Practical aspects of the instrumental management of tinnitus. British Journal of Audiology 19: 147–150
Spitzer J B, Goldstein B A, Salzbrenner LG, Mueller G 1983 Effect of tinnitus masker noise on speech discrimination in quiet and two noise backgrounds. Scandinavian Audiology 12: 197–200
Terry A M P, Jones D M, Davis B R, Slater R 1983 Parametric studies of tinnitus masking and residual inhibition. British Journal of Audiology 17: 245–256
Tewfik S 1984 Phonocephalography. An objective diagnosis of tinnitus. Journal of Laryngology 88: 869–874
Vernon J 1977 Attempts to relieve tinnitus. Journal of the American Auditory Society 2: 124–131
Vernon J, Schleuning A 1978 Tinnitus: a new management. Laryngoscope 88: 413–419
Vernon J A, Meikle M B 1981 Tinnitus masking: unresolved problems. In: Evered D, Lawrenson G (eds) Tinnitus. Ciba Foundation Symposium 85, Pitman, London, pp 239–262
Wilson H 1983 Vibratory massage of the middle ear by means of the telephone. New York Medical Journal 57: 221–222
Wilson J P 1980 Recording of the Kemp echo and tinnitus from the ear canal without averaging. Journal of Physiology 298: 8P–9P

6
K. I. Berliner and J. K. Cunningham

Tinnitus suppression in cochlear implantation

It is often the case in medicine that a discovery is really a rediscovery. One of the first few patients to receive the single-electrode cochlear implant at the House Ear Institute (HEI) in 1973 noted that, since wearing the implant, her tinnitus had totally disappeared. It did not reappear even when she turned her device off at night. The cochlear implant is an auditory prosthesis for the profoundly deaf that uses electrical current to stimulate the auditory nerve, producing a sensation of sound. The report by this patient aroused an interest at HEI in the possibility that electrical stimulation might also be used to relieve tinnitus. House et al (1976) went on to question their other patients who had had implants. Ten of 12 patients reported a reduction in tinnitus following cochlear implantation. The amount and quality of the reduction varied across patients, but was commonly related to a reduction in the number of characteristic sounds comprising the tinnitus.

As it turns out, the finding that electrical stimulation might help relieve tinnitus was explored in detail by Grapengiesser in a book published in 1801. Further, Hatton et al (1960) had studied the effects of galvanic current on tinnitus, using transcutaneous electrical stimulation. They found a positive effect in approximately 45% of their subjects.

Over the last decade, a number of researchers have begun to study the possibility of tinnitus suppression by means of electrical stimulation. Electrical currents have been applied with transcutaneous electrodes (Chouard et al 1981, Shulman 1985, Vernon & Fenwick 1985), transtympanic electrodes (Aran & Cazals 1981, Cazals et al 1978, Graham & Hazell 1977, Hazell et al 1985, House 1984, Portmann et al 1979), and intracochlear electrodes (Brackmann 1981, Pialoux et al 1979, Thedinger et al 1985). Transcutaneous electrodes have been used to explore the possibility of developing a noninvasive electrical treatment for tinnitus. Transtympanic electrodes have been placed both at the promontory and at the round window and have been used primarily for acute stimulation studies. Intracochlear electrodes have usually been implanted to restore hearing, although five patients were implanted for the express purpose of relieving their tinnitus (Thedinger et al 1985).

In addition to different electrode placements, different stimulus waveforms have been applied in these investigations. Portmann et al (1979), Chouard et al (1981), Aran & Cazals (1981), and Vernon & Fenwick (1985), in particular, report comparisons of the effects of a variety of stimuli including direct current pulses of different types and alternating current such as sine waves. Results, however, have been variable in terms of which stimulus is most effective.

The reported success rates in studies of the effects of electrical stimulation on tinnitus have also been highly variable, from as little as 20% to as high as 87%. 'Success' has usually been defined either as an all-or-none indication by the subject that the tinnitus has been suppressed or as a decrease in the severity of the tinnitus on a psychological scale. Despite the variability in success rate, every study has consistently found that at least some subjects had a reduction in their perceived tinnitus as a result of electrical stimulation.

The House Ear Institute has been involved in long-term clinical trials of the cochlear implant (House & Berliner 1982) and is therefore in a position to study the effects of chronic electrical stimulation on tinnitus. The remainder of this chapter is an in-depth look at the results from a tinnitus questionnaire used over a period of years at HEI, and, in particular, a careful examination of those findings of a clinical nature that might be useful for counselling patients regarding the possible effects of electrical stimulation on tinnitus and for determining prognosis for specific patients.

METHODS

Subjects

The subjects for this study were profoundly deaf adults who were participating in the clinical investigation of a single-electrode cochlear implant at the House Ear Institute or one of its co-investigator sites. All subjects had bilateral sensorineural deafness and had been selected to receive a cochlear implant for their primary complaint of hearing loss. A total of 130 subjects completed at least one post-implant tinnitus questionnaire and are included in some of the present analyses. However, most of the analyses were performed on a subset of the 130 implant patients. Characteristics of these subjects are presented in Table 6.1. Generally, they were older adults who had been deaf for an average of 13 years prior to receiving the cochlear implant. The sample of subjects included most of the aetiologies that produce a profound sensorineural hearing loss.

Table 6.1 Characteristics of subjects in the tinnitus study ($n=65$: 28 females (43%); 37 males (57%))

		No.	%
Use of hearing aid	Now	28	43
	In past	22	34
	Never	15	23
Aetiology ($n=62$)	Ototoxic	5	8.1
	Otosclerosis	14	22.6
	Meningitis	10	16.1
	Trauma	5	8.1
	Other	12	19.4
	Unknown	16	25.8

Mean age at onset of deafness: 35.5 years (SD=18.7)
Mean age at time of implant: 49.0 years (SD=15.0)

Materials

Data were collected by means of a tinnitus questionnaire completed by the subject. The questionnaire was based upon experience at HEI of tinnitus in profoundly deaf patients. It includes a description of the patient's tinnitus (e.g., check list of sounds heard, location, continuous vs. periodic, length of time an episode lasts); loudness and interference ratings; questions about what makes the tinnitus better and what makes it worse; previous treatments; and changes that have occurred over the years. The pre-implant version of the questionnaire asks whether a hearing aid affects the tinnitus and, if so, whether it makes it better or worse. The post-implant version asks whether the cochlear implant affects the tinnitus, and, if so, whether it makes the tinnitus better or worse.

In addition to the above, subjects completed a questionnaire on daily tinnitus and use of a prosthesis (hearing aid or implant). They rated the loudness and interference and noted hours of use of the device each day for a week. These rating scales were the same as the loudness and interference scales used on the tinnitus questionnaire. Definitions were provided to make ratings more consistent across subjects.
Loudness was rated as follows:

0 None—No head noise
1 Very soft—Heard only in a quiet situation
2 Moderate—Heard in an ordinary noise situation
3 Loud—Heard and noticed in all situations, even when concentrating on something else

Interference with daily life was rated as follows:

0 No interference—Causes no change in current activity
1 Slight interference—Can continue current activity but must go slower
2 Moderate interference—Cannot continue current activity but can perform a less demanding activity
3 Severe interference—Cannot perform any activity at all

Procedures

Subjects were asked to complete the pre-implant questionnaire prior to surgery for placement of the cochlear implant. (Note: Five subjects who already had implants at the beginning of this study completed the 'pre-implant' questionnaire retrospectively). They were again asked to complete the questionnaire approximately one year after the implant and annually thereafter. Subjects were also asked to complete the questionnaire on daily rating of tinnitus and use of device at regular follow-up intervals. Data from the pre-implant, initial post-implant, and the most recent post-implant questionnaires were analysed.

The stimulus received was that normally provided by the House cochlear implant signal processor: a 16 kHz sine wave, amplitude-modulated by the incoming speech and environmental sounds of daily life. When external sound was absent but the device was turned on, the 16 kHz signal was present at below-threshold levels. This device has been described in detail elsewhere (Danley & Fretz 1982).

RESULTS

Completed post-implant tinnitus questionnaires were obtained for a total of 130 subjects, independently of whether a subject had tinnitus before the implant. Of the 130, 40 (31%) had not experienced any tinnitus since they had last been asked, while 90 (69%) indicated that they had experienced tinnitus during the period in question. Of those 90, 48 (53%) stated that the cochlear implant made their tinnitus better, 32 (36%) felt that their tinnitus was unchanged by the implant, and 10 (11%) stated that their tinnitus was worse.

Seventy-three of the subjects had been in the study long enough to have filled in at least one questionnaire since the initial post-implant one. This provided the opportunity to examine whether there was any change in the effect of the implant on tinnitus over time. The mean time interval between the initial questionnaire and the most recent one was 13 months (range 2 to 25). Of the 73 subjects, 53 (73%) reported having tinnitus at the time of the initial questionnaire. Fifty-two (71%) of them reported tinnitus on the most recent questionnaire. Of the 53 subjects reporting tinnitus on the initial questionnaire, 36 (68%) felt that the implant made their tinnitus better, 13 (25%) felt that their tinnitus was unaffected, and 4 (8%) felt that their tinnitus was worse. On the most recent questionnaire, these numbers are: 37 (70%) better, 13 (25%) unaffected, and 3 (6%) who stated 'worse' on at least one follow-up.

In no case was the difference between the initial and the most recent responses statistically significant. That is, those subjects who felt after the initial post-implant interval that the implant had helped their tinnitus still felt so an average of one year later. Those whose tinnitus was initially unaffected by the implant continued to feel so. Finally, a small number of subjects continued to feel that the implant made their tinnitus worse. The questionnaires from all subjects who indicated that the cochlear implant made their tinnitus worse were examined in detail. Comments written on the questionnaires by the subjects, or inconsistent responses on later questionnaires, indicated that very few subjects actually felt that the implant had a significant negative impact on their tinnitus.

The results noted above are based solely on the subjects' responses to the post-implant tinnitus questionnaire item on whether the implant affected tinnitus. A detailed analysis of other responses on both pre-implant and most recent post-implant questionnaires was performed on a smaller group of subjects for whom these data were available. Not all subjects answered all questions: therefore, the number of subjects (n) in each analysis varies: the maximum was 71. Forty-eight subjects completed both pre-and post-implant questionnaires and answered the question regarding the effect of the implant on their tinnitus. On the average, the most recent questionnaires were completed 17 months post-implant (range 6 months to 10 years). Following is a summary description of the tinnitus experienced by these subjects, an analysis of the effects of the implant on tinnitus, and an analysis of predictive indices.

Tinnitus characteristics

Since the sample of subjects in this study—profoundly deaf adults— represents a population of tinnitus sufferers not frequently described, the characteristics of their tinnitus are presented here in some detail. Fifty-two of them reported the length of time they had experienced tinnitus: the average was 16 years, although the variability between subjects was high (SD=12.6). About half of the subjects in the study had continuous tinnitus ($n=30$), the other half periodic ($n=32$). The location of tinnitus was the right ear for 10 (16%) of the subjects, the left ear for 6 (10%), both ears for 24 (39%), and was not localized for 21 (34%).

To assess the kinds of noises experienced, each subject was asked whether he/she experienced any of 15 specific sounds: buzzing, roaring, clicking, high-pitched ringing, low-pitched ringing, whooshing, hissing, cricket-like sound, pounding, pulsating, whistle, steam whistle, bells, clanging, and 'other'. Of these noises, the most frequently occurring were buzzing ($n=42$ of 62; 68%), roaring ($n=40$; 65%), clicking ($n=22$; 36), and low-pitched ringing ($n=19$; 31%). Each of the remaining noises was experienced by fewer than 30% of the 62 subjects. The mean number of noises experienced by the group of subjects was 4.7 (SD=3.0).

Fifty-seven subjects rated the loudness of their tinnitus: 21 (37%) reported it as loud, 24 (42%) as moderate, and 12 (21%) as soft.

When asked about the extent to which tinnitus interfered with their daily lives, 38 (62%) of 61 subjects reported that it did not interfere. Fifteen (25%) reported that it interfered slightly; 7 (12%) reported moderate interference; and one reported that it was a severe problem.

Various factors may influence an individual's tinnitus. To help identify these, subjects were asked to indicate whether or not each of 17 naturally and/or commonly occurring factors (Table 6.2) made their tinnitus worse. Two of the factors—fatigue and nervousness—negatively affected 40% or more of the 57 subjects who responded. Another six factors—excitement, physical activity, worry, noisy places, change in weather, and lack of sleep—each affected over 20%. It appears that tinnitus can be negatively influenced by a wide range of factors.

Table 6.2 Number and percentage of 57 subjects who indicated their tinnitus was made worse by given factors

Factors	n	%
Fatigue	29	51
Excitement	16	28
Physical activity	15	26
Lack of sleep	12	21
Constipation	2	4
Head or body positions	7	12
Exposure to loud sounds	11	19
Noisy places	13	23
Nervousness	23	40
Change in weather	13	23
Aspirin	4	7
Worry	13	23
Medication	1	2
Menstrual periods	6	11
Alcohol	1	2
Anger	9	16
Other	6	11

Just as everyday factors can aggravate tinnitus, some may help relieve tinnitus. Subjects were asked whether or not each of nine factors made their tinnitus better. As shown in Table 6.3, only two of the nine factors—sleep and rest—affected a substantial percentage of the people in this sample.

Table 6.3 Number and percentage of 57 subjects who indicated their tinnitus was helped by given factors

Factors	n	%
Sleep	36	63
Food	2	4
Sedative	2	4
Tranquillizer	8	14
Alcohol	0	0
Rest	23	40
Exercise	3	5
Relaxation techniques	3	5
Other	11	19

In addition to 'everyday' influences on tinnitus, many of the subjects in this study felt that their pre-implant prostheses—hearing aids—affected their tinnitus. Fifty-three people in the study sample wore or had worn a hearing aid. Of these, 24 (45%) reported that the aid affected their tinnitus. Two subjects did not indicate whether the hearing aid made their tinnitus better or worse. Of the remaining 22, 13 (59%) indicated that the aid made their tinnitus better, while 9 (41%) reported the opposite. It appears that hearing aids positively affected only about one-fourth (13 of 53) of those who wore a hearing aid.

The effect of the cochlear implant on tinnitus

As noted earlier, 53% of 90 subjects with tinnitus for whom the results of post-implant tinnitus questionnaires were available felt that the implant affected their tinnitus for the better. In the present analyses, 35 (49%) of the 71 subjects who rated the effect of the implant on their tinnitus indicated that the implant made their tinnitus better. Twenty-nine (41%) of the 71 subjects indicated that the implant had no effect, and 7 (10%) reported that the implant made their tinnitus worse.

Those who indicated that the implant had an effect were asked to indicate whether any of five possible characteristics of the tinnitus had changed. As seen in Table 6.4, the effect of the implant differed in different individuals. Each of the listed characteristics was selected by no more than about one-third of the 29 subjects who answered this question and who reported that the implant made their tinnitus better. A similar pattern occurred for those who indicated that the implant made their tinnitus worse, although the small number of such subjects makes the percentages more varied.

Sixty-four subjects reported which ear was affected by the implant. Of these, only 14% indicated the implanted ear, 13% indicated the other ear, 52% indicated both ears, and the remaining 22% could not localize the effect. Unfortunately, 24 subjects who indicated that the implant had no effect on their tinnitus went on and answered

Table 6.4 Number and percentage of subjects reporting a change in each of five tinnitus characteristics for those whose tinnitus was made better ($n=29$) or worse ($n=6$) by the implant

	Implant effect on tinnitus			
Tinnitus	Better		Worse	
characteristics	n	%	n	%
Loudness	10	35	3	50
No. of different sounds	8	28	4	67
Frequency of occurrence	9	31	1	17
Pitch of the sounds	4	14	1	17
Duration of noises	4	14	1	17

the question regarding which ear was affected! Perhaps it was not clear that this question referred only to the effect of the implant on tinnitus. However, if one looks at the responses from only those subjects ($n=34$) who indicated that the implant improved their tinnitus, the percentage noting an effect on both ears was 56%. Similarly, of the few subjects who felt that the implant made their tinnitus worse, 3 out of 6 (50%) indicated that both ears were affected.

In addition to asking subjects whether or not they felt that the implant affected their tinnitus, a number of 'measures' of tinnitus were obtained from both the pre-implant and post-implant questionnaires. Significant changes are discussed below. The relationship between the subjects' ratings of effect and changes in these other measures is also examined. Three measures were assessed: 1. differences in loudness; 2. differences in number and type of noises; and 3. differences in the degree to which tinnitus interferes with daily life.

Before turning to these analyses, it should be noted that of 65 subjects who reported having tinnitus during the year before implantation, all but 13 (20%) reported that they had experienced tinnitus during the period after implantation. It is not clear whether the implant eliminated head noise for the 13 subjects who did not report post-implant tinnitus, or whether some other factor was involved. Information on whether or not the tinnitus was periodic or continuous before the implant was available for 12 of the 13 subjects. Nine (75%) of those 12 had indicated that their tinnitus was periodic. Given that about half of the subjects in this study had periodic tinnitus, a binominal test indicates that the likelihood of finding that nine or more of these 12 subjects had periodic tinnitus is only 0.07, just short of statistical significance. This suggests that the reports of no post-implant tinnitus may be due in part to periodicity of the tinnitus. On the other hand, the time period involved is such that one would not expect even periodic tinnitus to remain 'off' for that duration. At any rate, these 13 subjects are not included in any of the following analyses.

Loudness

Subjects were asked before and after the implant to rate the loudness of the tinnitus in their left ear, right ear, and head according to the four-point scale described earlier.

Median ratings from the pre-and post-implant daily tinnitus questionnaires were obtained. This resulted in six ratings; three pre-test and three post-test. The most extreme (loudest) of the three pre-test scores and the most extreme of the three post-test scores, regardless of ear, were then retained for analysis of change in loudness. A paired comparison t-test was used to assess the difference between these highest pre- and post-implant ratings. The mean difference was statistically significant ($t_{39} = -3.79, p < 0.001$). Post-implant loudness ratings (mean=0.80) were lower than pre-implant loudness ratings (mean=1.33).

The change in loudness was then compared to the ratings of the effect of the cochlear implant (i.e. Better, Worse, No Effect). Data from 25 subjects were available for this analysis. These are shown in Table 6.5. Thirteen subjects experienced a reduction in loudness and 12 did not. Of those that experienced a reduction, the majority (62%) reported that the implant had a positive effect. Of the subjects who experienced no reduction in loudness, the majority (67%) reported that the implant had no effect.

Table 6.5 Relationship between change in loudness of the tinnitus and rated effect of the implant ($n = 25$)

Loudness	Implant effect			
	Better	No effect	Worse	Total
Reduced	8 (62%)	4 (31%)	1 (8%)	13
No change	3 (25%)	8 (67%)	1 (8%)	12

Sixteen of the 25 subjects in this analysis had loudness scores that were consistent with their assessment of the effect of the cochlear implant. However, a chi-squared test of the association between the change in loudness scores and the implant ratings did not indicate a significant relationship (chi-squared=2.17, $p=0.14$, using Better and No Effect cells only).

Number and type of noises

Pre- and post-implant measures of the 15 noises described earlier were used to analyse the difference between the number of pre-implant noises and the number of post-implant noises experienced by the subjects as tinnitus. Results indicated a statistically significant decrease in the number of noises (Wilcoxon matched-pairs signed-ranks test: $Z=-1.62, p<0.05$). On the average, subjects ($n=47$) experienced 5.1 noises before the implant and 4.4 noises after the implant.

To examine the relationship between ratings of the effect of the cochlear implant and decreases in number of noises experienced from pre- to post-implant, Wilcoxon's matched-pairs signed-ranks test was again used to assess whether or not the distribution of pre-implant noises differed significantly from the distribution of post-implant noises. However, this time the analysis was based on the rating of effect of implant on tinnitus.

For those subjects who reported a positive implant effect ($n=22$), there was a statistically significant decrease in the number of noises ($Z=-1.71, p<0.05$). On the average, these subjects had 5.0 different noises before the implant and 3.9 noises after the implant. For those subjects who reported no effect of the implant on tinnitus ($n=18$), the difference in pre- and post-implant noises was not statistically significant ($Z=-0.75$, $p=0.20$). They averaged 5.0 noises pre-implant and 4.2 noises post-implant. This analysis suggests that the ratings of implant effect may be associated with changes in number of tinnitus noises experienced.

Pre- and post-implant measures of the 15 noises were further analysed using the McNemar test for correlated proportions to determine whether or not particular noises were more likely to stop after the implant. Table 6.6 presents the number and percentage of subjects indicating presence of each noise pre- and post-implant. A statistically significant decrease in those reporting buzzing was found. Thirteen of 34 subjects reporting buzzing pre-implant did not do so post-implant. None of the other noises showed statistically significant decreases.

Table 6.6 Number and percentage of 50 subjects experiencing each of 15 noises as tinnitus pre-implant and post-implant

	Pre-implant		Post-implant	
Noises	n	%	n	%
Buzzing	34	68	23	46
Roaring	34	68	34	68
Clicking	19	38	19	38
High-pitched ringing	26	52	20	40
Low-pitched ringing	19	38	17	34
Whooshing	14	28	14	28
Hissing	15	30	12	24
Cricket-like	16	32	12	24
Pounding	7	14	11	22
Pulsating	10	20	9	18
Whistle	13	26	12	24
Steam whistle	8	16	5	10
Bells	12	24	8	16
Clanging	10	20	6	12
Other ($n=47$)	12	26	11	23

To assess whether or not the rating of the effect of the implant was associated with the presence or absence of particular noises, pre- and post-implant scores for the 15 noises were analysed using a series of McNemar tests as before. This time, however, the tests were run separately for those subjects ($n=23$) who rated the implant positively and those ($n=20$) who rated the implant as having no effect. None of the results proved statistically significant. Thus there was no evidence to suggest that the post-implant absence of a given noise is associated with ratings of the effect of the implant on tinnitus.

Amount of interference

Whether there was a change in how much the subjects' tinnitus interfered with their daily lives was examined by comparing the pre- and post-implant interference ratings. A Wilcoxon test showed a statistically significant difference between pre- and post-implant ($n=40$, $Z=-2.19$, $p<0.01$). The mean interference ratings pre- and post-implant were 0.38 and 0.15, respectively. Of the 40 subjects, 8 had lower interference ratings post-implant than pre-implant, one had a higher rating post-implant than pre-implant, and 31 had no change.

Differences in the degree to which tinnitus interferes with daily life before and after the implant may be associated with how subjects rate the effect of the implant. Further analysis showed that of six subjects who had a decrease in interference from pre-implant to post-implant and who rated the effect of the implant, three reported that the implant made their tinnitus better, two reported that the implant made their tinnitus worse, and one reported that the implant had no effect. These data do not indicate that the amount of interference affected the subjects' rating of the effect of the implant on tinnitus.

Prognostic indicators

The ability to predict which patients may obtain tinnitus relief from the cochlear implant is of importance to the clinician. An analysis of the relationship between aetiology of hearing loss and whether the implant helped tinnitus was performed for all subjects whose aetiology was a known cause and who had completed at least one post-implant questionnaire. Responses from the most recent questionnaire were used. Aetiologies included ototoxic, otosclerosis, meningitis, trauma, and 'other'. The proportion of subjects reporting improvement in tinnitus was compared to that reporting no change or worsening. No statistically significant relationship between aetiology and effect of the implant on tinnitus was found ($n=114$, chi-squared=1.72, $p=0.5$).

In addition to looking at aetiology, we analysed many of the items on the pre-implant tinnitus questionnaire in relation to whether the subjects rated the implant as affecting their tinnitus for the better (score=1), no effect (score=2), or for the worse (score=3).

A series of t-tests was performed to assess possible associations between the rating of the effect of the cochlear implant and those factors that subjects noted as making their tinnitus worse. Results are presented in Table 6.7. Fatigue, noisy places, and nervousness had statistically significant relationships with assessment of the implant. Subjects whose tinnitus was affected by fatigue and nervousness tended to feel that the implant helped their tinnitus. Subjects whose tinnitus was affected by noisy places tended to feel that the implant had no effect on their tinnitus.

Of the eight factors described earlier that may positively influence head noise, only – sleep and rest – affected more than a few people. These two factors did not have statistically significant associations with ratings of the effect of the implant ($t_{42}=-0.75$, $p=0.46$ and $t_{42}=-0.87$, $p=0.39$, respectively).

For the 15 noises used to describe tinnitus, t-tests were performed to explore whether or not the pre-implant presence of a given noise was associated with the effect of the implant. Statistically significant associations were not found, although the test result for 'cricket-like' sounds approached significance ($t_{44}=-1.81$, $p<0.08$). The mean cochlear implant rating for people who experienced cricket-like sounds was 1.3, and that for those who did not experience such sounds was 1.7; that is, those whose

Table 6.7 Mean rating of the effect of the implant on tinnitus in 43 subjects whose tinnitus was adversely affected by given factors

Factors	Affected by factor	Not affected by factor	t value
Fatigue	1.3	1.9	−3.81[2]
Excitement	1.4	1.7	−1.56
Physical activity	1.6	1.5	.32
Lack of sleep	1.5	1.6	−.69
Head or body positions	1.8	1.5	1.12
Exposure to loud sounds	1.9	1.5	1.56
Noisy places	1.9	1.5	1.97[1]
Nervousness	1.3	1.8	−2.75[2]
Change in weather	1.7	1.5	.64
Worry	1.5	1.6	−.69
Anger	1.3	1.6	−1.62

[1] $p<0.05$ [2] $p<0.01$
The rating scale used was: 1 = positive effect of implant, 2 = no effect, 3 = negative effect

tinnitus was described as including a 'cricket-like' sound were slightly more likely to feel that the implant made their tinnitus better.

Whether the tinnitus was periodic or continuous did not prove to be a statistically significant predictor of the implant's effect ($t_{44}=-1.30$, $p=0.20$). Subjects with continuous head noise had a mean rating of 1.5. Those with periodic head noise had a mean of 1.7.

Finally, an analysis of subjects who reported that their hearing aids affected their tinnitus before their implant indicated that subjects tended to rate the implant positively (mean=1.18) if their hearing aids positively affected their tinnitus. They tended to rate the effect of the implant on tinnitus less positively (mean=2.5) if their hearing aids worsened their tinnitus. This difference was statistically significant ($t_{13}=-5.01$, $p<0.01$).

DISCUSSION

The present study examined tinnitus suppression by chronic electrical stimulation through use of a cochlear implant. The subjects were profoundly deaf adults implanted for the purpose of auditory stimulation. They represent, therefore, a fairly specific population of individuals who may experience tinnitus. Approximately 53% of these subjects indicated that the cochlear implant had a positive effect on their tinnitus. This finding is consistent with previous findings and indicates that electrical stimulation may offer an avenue of treatment for at least some tinnitus sufferers.

Subjects who indicated that the implant helped their tinnitus varied in what they felt had changed about their tinnitus. Loudness, number of different sounds heard, frequency of occurrence of tinnitus, pitch of the sounds, or length of time the noises last per episode were each improved for at least some of the subjects.

For the subjects as a group, there were significant reductions in the loudness of the tinnitus from pre-implant to post-implant, the amount of interference, and the number of different sounds experienced. House et al (1976) had also reported a reduction in the number of sounds experienced as tinnitus post-implant.

Changes in ratings of loudness, number and type of sounds, and amount of interference from pre- to post-implant were not always consistent with whether the subject rated his/her tinnitus as improved by the implant. This is not too surprising given the complex interactions possible among all of the factors affecting tinnitus.

There was a significant relationship between whether or not a hearing aid had ever helped reduce the subjects' tinnitus and whether the implant helped. This finding is especially interesting in the light of Shulman's (1985) observation that most of his subjects who achieved tinnitus suppression with transcutaneous electrical stimulation were also able to have their tinnitus masked.

Subjects who felt that fatigue-like or stress-related factors made their tinnitus worse were more likely to have an improvement with the implant. Deaf adults who have received the cochlear implant often comment that they experience a reduction in the attention and concentration required for successful communication, and therefore less fatigue. By reducing fatigue, the implant may indirectly affect tinnitus. This would be consistent with the finding that tinnitus in both ears was affected by the implant for some subjects, even though they received a cochlear implant in only one ear. On the other hand, this stress reduction mechanism would not easily account for the 'residual inhibition' seen in many of the implant subjects. Even when not wearing their implant device, the subjects' tinnitus may remain absent for hours or days. For instance, in the first patient to report the effect of the implant on her tinnitus (House et al 1976), the tinnitus remained suppressed for more than two weeks when her device was not functioning, before it began to return. Thus, for some subjects the implant effect may be stress reduction, for some it may be a form of tinnitus masking, and for some a true suppression.

Variables other than those just discussed were not generally predictive of effects of cochlear implantation on tinnitus. For example, there was no evidence that the aetiology of the hearing loss was related to the impact of the implant on tinnitus.

Among the interesting aspects of this study must be noted the complexity of the questionnaire data. Subjects were not always consistent in their responses, and often they did not answer all questions. This created numerous methodological problems when analysing the data, including the distracting problem of constantly changing numbers of subjects (n). However, this probably reflects the very real complexity of the symptom—tinnitus—under study.

The present study examined subjects who received a cochlear implant for a reason other than tinnitus suppression. A recent study, however, reported findings on a small number of subjects who were implanted specifically for the indication of severe tinnitus (Thedinger et al 1985). These were patients for whom all other treatments had proven ineffective. In only one of the five cases was the result considered a definite success. This was a patient who had a progressive hearing loss of unknown aetiology with a sudden onset of tinnitus. Three of the remaining patients were undergoing a vestibular nerve section for severe vertigo, and the cochlear implant was placed during the same surgical procedure. It may be that these particular types of cases do not have a good prognosis for tinnitus suppression by electrical stimulation.

In all, the present results indicate that some profoundly deaf patients may obtain relief from tinnitus by use of the cochlear implant. Furthermore, a few clinical factors were related to the occurrence of such relief. Still needed are a better understanding of the mechanisms underlying the effects of the cochlear implant on tinnitus and a better definition of those variables that might enable accurate prediction of such effects.

REFERENCES

Aran J-M, Cazals Y 1981 Electrical suppression of tinnitus. In: Evered D, Lawrenson G (eds) Tinnitus. Ciba Foundation Symposium 85. Pitman, London, pp 217–231
Brackmann D E 1981 Reduction of tinnitus in cochlear implant patients. In: Proceedings of the First International Tinnitus Seminar, New York. Journal of Laryngology and Otology Supplement 4: 163–165
Cazals Y, Negrevergne M, Aran J-M 1978 Electrical stimulation of the cochlea in man: Hearing inducation and tinnitus suppression. Journal of the American Audiology Society 3: 209–213
Chouard C-H, Meyer B, Maridat D 1981 Transcutaneous electrotherapy for severe tinnitus. Acta Otolaryngologica 91: 415–422
Danley M J, Fretz R J 1982 Design and functioning of the single-electrode cochlear implant. In: House W F, Berliner K I (eds) Cochlear implants: progress and perspectives. Annals of Otology, Rhinology, and Laryngology 91 (Supplement 91): 21–26
Graham J M, Hazell J W P 1977 Electrical stimulation of the human cochlea using a transtympanic electrode. British Journal of Audiology 11: 59–62
Grapengiesser C J C 1801 Versuche den Galvanismus zur Heilung einiger Krankheiten (Berlin). Cited in: Feldmann H 1984 Suppression of tinnitus by electrical stimulation: A contribution to the history of medicine. In: Proceedings of the Second International Tinnitus Seminar, New York, 1983. Journal of Laryngology and Otology, Supplement 9: 123–124
Hatton D S, Erulkar S D, Rosenberg P E 1960 Some preliminary observations on the effect of galvanic current on tinnitus aurium. Laryngoscope 70: 123–130
Hazell J W P, Graham J M, Rothera M P 1985 Electrical stimulation of the cochlea and tinnitus. In: Schindler R A, Merzenich M M (eds) Cochlear implants. Raven Press, New York, pp 563–568
House J W 1984 Effects of electrical stimulation on tinnitus. In: Proceedings of the Second International Tinnitus Seminar, New York, 1983. Journal of Laryngology and Otology, Supplement 9: 139–140
House W F, Berliner K I 1982 Cochlear implants: progress and perspectives. Annals of Otology, Rhinology, and Laryngology 91 (Supplement 91): 1–124
House W F, Berliner K I, Crary W G et al 1976 Cochlear implants. Annals of Otology, Rhinology, and Laryngology 85 (Supplement 27): 1–93
Pialoux P, Chouard C H, Meyer B, Fugain C 1979 Indications and results of the multichannel cochlear implant. Acta Oto-laryngologica 87: 185–189
Portmann M, Cazals Y, Negrevergne M, Aran J-M 1979 Temporary tinnitus suppression in man through electrical stimulation of the cochlea. Acta Oto-laryngologica 87: 294–299
Shulman A 1985 External electrical stimulation in tinnitus control. American Journal of Otology 6: 110–115
Thedinger B, House W F, Edgerton B J 1985 Cochlear implant for tinnitus–case reports. Annals of Otology, Rhinology, and Laryngology 94: 10–13
Vernon J A, Fenwick J A 1985 Attempts to suppress tinnitus with transcutaneous electrical stimulation. Otolaryngology 93: 385–389

7 *J. M. Graham*

Tinnitus in hearing-impaired children

'Deaf children don't get tinnitus' (folklore)

'These (deaf) children have enough problems; if you draw their attention to tinnitus, you'll only make them worse' (Headmaster, School for the Deaf)

Children are remarkably tolerant. Few children with a 30 dB hearing loss imposed by glue ear actually complain about it. It is not surprising that in 1979 some preliminary telephone calls to teachers of the deaf and to paediatric audiologists produced the reply that deaf children did not seem to have tinnitus; the exceptions were thought to be a few, often rather odd, cases, such as the child with objective tonal tinnitus described by Glanville et al (1971). The suggestion that a congenitally deaf child, with no auditory memory, would not recognise tinnitus (even if the physiological events normally associated, in adults, with 'subjective' tinnitus were present) was supported by this report, since the child in question had tinnitus audible by onlookers at a distance of several yards but could not hear it himself.

Nodar (1972) seems to have been the first author to look at the prevalence of tinnitus in children. In a survey of 2000 school children aged 11 to 18 (5th to 12th school grades) 15% reported that they had tinnitus. However the duration and severity of the tinnitus was not reported. Since in adults tinnitus usually occurs in association with a hearing loss (Coles 1984) it seemed likely that if any children with tinnitus existed they should be concentrated in schools for the hearing-impaired. In the United Kingdom the majority of deaf children (those with deafness requiring hearing aids) attend special Partial Hearing Units (PHUs) attached to ordinary schools. Schools for the deaf, with no normally hearing pupils, are generally reserved for the most profoundly deaf and those with very poor spoken language, particularly when they have other disabilities or social problems. In 1979, in spite of the fact that teachers of the deaf had told me, informally, that in their view few of the children in their care had tinnitus, I approached the head teachers of the PHUs of the Inner London Education Authority, scattered in a wide circle north and south of the river Thames. They kindly agreed to carry out a survey of the 12–18-year-olds in their schools. This is the secondary school age in England and seemed the most likely to give reliable answers to questions.

132 TINNITUS

LONDON SURVEY RESULTS

The first survey (Graham 1981a) was of 74 children from five PHUs. The main findings were:

1. 64% of the children had tinnitus.
2. Only two children had continuous tinnitus: in the rest it was intermittent.
3. In the small number (14) who had a hearing loss symmetrical between the two ears and unilateral aiding, the tinnitus was equally distributed between the aided and the unaided ears, so was not consistently related to the use of aids.
4. Tinnitus was commoner in a child's better hearing ear.
5. The degree of annoyance was considered to be disturbing in 40% of the children.

The findings from this initial survey were interesting enough to lead to a second, more detailed study (Graham 1981b) in which the same five PHUs were approached, together with two schools for the deaf. The original set of questions was asked, with a supplementary list of more detailed questions (see Appendix 7.1) designed to find out how long the tinnitus lasted, how often it occurred, how loud it was, whether it impaired hearing and whether it was accompanied by other symptoms such as vertigo (Snashall 1984).

The questions in the survey were sent to the schools. Class teachers identified children with tinnitus by direct questioning, distributed the lists of questions to all these children and made sure that each child understood the questions. They also sent the author a copy of each child's audiogram, details of aids worn, and the medical diagnosis of the supposed cause of deafness, where known. In the schools for the deaf there was some selection of pupils: the teachers did not include those children with very poor language, who might not have understood the questions asked. All 78 children who said they had tinnitus were asked the general questions shown in Appendix 7.1. A smaller group of 48 children (29 in PHUs, 19 in schools for the deaf) were asked the more detailed questions shown in the second part of Appendix 7.1. As expected, the average hearing thresholds (250, 500, 1000 and 2000 Hz nHL in the better hearing ear) were worse in children from schools for the deaf (95 dB) than in the PHUs (52.5 dB).

Prevalence of tinnitus

The prevalence of tinnitus in the whole group of 158 children was 49%, lower than in the first study. This is because the schools for the deaf reported a lower incidence (only 29%) than the PHUs (66%) (Table 7.1). Both Reich (1981) and Nodar (1984)

Table 7.1 Prevalence of tinnitus among children at partial-hearing units (PHUs) and schools for the deaf (Schools)

	Total	PHUs	Schools
Number of children questioned	158	92	66
Number who had tinnitus	78 (49%)	59 (66%)	19 (29%)

have examined the prevalence of tinnitus in deaf children and report similar figures. Reich circulated children in Portland, Oregon, and received replies from 46 children of whom 18 reported that they had tinnitus. The tinnitus was intermittent in all but two. Nodar collected data from 56 deaf children in Cleveland, Ohio, and found a 55% incidence of tinnitus. Again only two children had constant tinnitus.

Tinnitus and degree of hearing loss

The prevalence of tinnitus in the PHUs was twice as high as in the schools for the deaf. This might be directly related to the better hearing of the PHU children (Table 7.2) particularly since, of those with unilateral tinnitus who had a difference in hearing (10 dB or more, average threshold difference) between their two ears, most (80%) had the tinnitus in their *better* ear. Nodar & Lezak (1984) also found a lower incidence (35%) of tinnitus in more profoundly deaf children (70-110 dB) than in those with better hearing (50-70 dB) and those with a high-frequency loss only. The last two groups had, in the rather small number (18) assessed, a 100% prevalence of tinnitus. It seems that deaf children with better hearing are more likely to have tinnitus; a possible reason was proposed by Kemp (1981) who suggested that because the quality of sounds perceived by the profoundly deaf is so poor, they may not be able to distinguish between endogenous tinnitus and the distorted sound sensations they receive from their environment. This factor could be linked, in children with poor spoken language and verbal reasoning, with the difficulty of conveying to them the concept of tinnitus. Emmett (1981) said that he had the same problem when trying to find out whether children under the age of six had tinnitus. Conceptual difficulties (a rose by any other name...) are not confined to children. With recent publicity about tinnitus clinicians have become familiar with patients with noises in their ears who say 'I hope it's not that tinnitus thing I've read about.' Molière's M. Jourdain had the same problem: 'ma foi! il y a plus de quarante ans que je dis la prose sans que j'en susse rien. (Good God! D'you mean I've been talking prose for forty years without knowing it?)'

Table 7.2 Average hearing thresholds (dB HL) of children with tinnitus

	250 Hz	500 Hz	1 kHz	2 kHz
Children in partial-hearing units				
(PHUs) ($n=59$)	42 dB	50	55	63
Range	(5–110 dB)	(5–110)	(10–110)	(10–110)
Children in schools for the deaf				
(Schools) ($n=19$)	79	91	102	108
Range	(60–90)	(75–105)	(80–120)	(80–120)

The prevalence of tinnitus seems to have been much higher than expected by those adults who teach deaf children. Goodey (1981) observed that most of the members of a club for young congenitally deaf adults told him that they had tinnitus. Very few deaf children with tinnitus complain about the symptom, in contrast with the suffering experienced by adults who had acquired tinnitus. However if children seldom complain about tinnitus this does not, as will be seen later, mean that the symptom is never troublesome. The severity of deafness is not the only factor related to tinnitus in deaf children. In some the use of a hearing aid may be relevant. Aids have a masking effect on tinnitus in some adults and may do so in children; this explains why many children commented that the tinnitus appeared when they removed their aids (Graham & Butler 1984); however in at least two children the tinnitus was clearly *provoked* by aid use. Any possible interaction between the better hearing ear and unilateral aiding was not, unfortunately, clarified by the survey: there was a group of 15 children with both tinnitus and a unilateral aid in their better hearing ear, but this simply reflects the current practice of fitting single aids in better ears.

Intermittent *vs.* constant tinnitus

An interesting contrast is between constant and intermittent tinnitus. In adults with acquired tinnitus the symptom is usually constant (Hazell 1981, Coles et al 1981). In congenitally deaf children this seems to be extremely rara (Table 7.3). Nodar & Le Zak (1984) and Reich (1981) reported similar findings. It is possible that where the physiological activity associated with tinnitus is present in a steady state from birth, it may not be perceived. Attempts have been made to define 'subclinical' or unperceived tinnitus. If this rather dubious concept had any value it would be as a description of such a physiological steady state in children.

Table 7.3 Frequency with which tinnitus occurred

Frequency of tinnitus	Numbers of children		
	Total	PHUs	Schools
Constant	2	0	2
Daily	9	5	4
More than 3 times a week	7	6	1
1–3 times a week	13	7	6
Monthly	6	5	1
Less often	11	7	4
Number of replies:	48	30	18

Aetiology of deafness

In speculating about the site of origin of tinnitus in those born deaf, rather than deprived of hearing, it would have been interesting if certain recognised causes of deafness in which the histopathology is known, were more likely to produce tinnitus. The two surveys reported here (Graham 1981a, b) used data from class teachers, not doctors. The diagnoses listed in Table 7.4 include a large number of children where the cause of deafness was unknown or not recorded, and the 'hereditary deafness' group was not analysed. The diagnosis was only recorded in those children who had tinnitus, so no comparison could be made between tinnitus and non-tinnitus children.

Secretory otitis media is a common cause of tinnitus but has a relatively low prevalence in older children. 30% of the children in the surveys said that they had ear

Table 7.4 List of diagnoses

Numbers of children	
Partial-hearing units	Schools for the deaf
11 Hereditary deafness	4 Hereditary deafness
7 Anoxia	3 Meningitis
6 Congenital middle-ear abnormality	1 Anoxia
5 Rubella	1 Rubella
3 Chronic infective ear disease	10 Unknown
2 Serous otitis media	
2 Meningitis	
2 Measles	
1 Rickets (?)	
22 Unknown	

infections, glue ear, myringotomies, or grommet insertion at some time: this figure is around average for the general population. The survey did not establish how many of the children had secretory otitis media or grommets at the time the questions were answered; it seems likely that among 12–18-year-olds in the month of June the prevalence of secretory otitis media would have been low. A few children were known to have either congenital middle ear deformities or chronic suppurative otitis media (Table 7.4).

Symptoms that may accompany tinnitus

Many of the spontaneous comments of the children in the first survey (Graham 1981a) drew attention to specific problems produced by tinnitus. Several children said that they felt dizzy when they had tinnitus. In the more detailed second survey (Graham 1981b) 22 of the 78 children said that they felt dizzy on some occasions with the tinnitus (Table 7.5). Allowing for the natural eagerness of children to give positive answers to direct questions, and for the failure to clarify what was meant by dizziness, this is quite a large population. Snashall (1984) points out that vertigo, like tinnitus, is a relatively unrecognised problem in children. It is likely that some of the children in the survey may have had endolymphatic hydrops: this can certainly occur with the Mondini deformity (Illum 1972). Vertiginous epilepsy in children may be accompanied by tinnitus (Alpers 1960) but is not particularly associated with congenital deafness. Perilymph leak can occur in congenitally deaf children and is

Table 7.5 Incidence of dizziness or headache accompanying the tinnitus

	Numbers of children		
Symptom	Total	PHUs	Schools
Number with accompanying dizziness	22 (46%)	16 (55%)	6 (32%)
Number with accompanying headache	11 (23%)	6 (20%)	5 (26%)
Number of replies:	48	29	19

Percentages are of total number of replies in each column.

associated with tinnitus and vertigo; however, none of the children in either survey was known to have a perilymph leak.

Headache seemed to be another symptom that occurred with tinnitus (Table 7.5). Apart from specific reasons for headache such as discomfort from recruitment and migrainous episodes, headache suggests the presence of some stress generated by annoying tinnitus.

Troublesome tinnitus

The degree of annoyance caused by tinnitus is notoriously difficult to assess. Different aspects of tinnitus cause distress to different people. Among adults there are those for whom tinnitus in the quiet of the evening is particularly trying, while others can get to sleep easily enough but are plagued anew by head noises as soon as they wake. Anxiety and stress make one man's tinnitus loud, but in another, divert attention from it. A patient may complain bitterly about tinnitus that is eventually found by matching and masking to be equivalent to less than 5 dB sensation level. It is hard, therefore, to find a satisfactory method of assessing the annoyance that tinnitus causes in a child. In the surveys I used four arbitrary criteria: those children who had tinnitus every day, had tinnitus lasting more than 30 minutes at a time, graded their tinnitus as 'very loud' on a scale of three degrees of loudness, and, on the assumption that annoyance is in the mind of the beholder, graded it at the highest of four grades of annoyance (Tables 7.3, 7.6, 7.7, 7.8). It seemed reasonable to include children who said that they had vertigo or headaches or who cried whenever the tinnitus was present. These criteria produced a group of one-third (31%) of the children with tinnitus which could be said to be annoying (Table 7.9). Since in 1982

Table 7.6 Duration of tinnitus

Duration	Numbers of children		
	Total	PHUs	Schools
Tinnitus for <5 min at a time:	23 (48%)	13 (41%)	10 (48%)
Tinnitus for >5 min at a time:	25 (52%)	17 (59%)	8 (42%)
Of these, tinnitus for >30 min at a time:	10 (21%)	7 (24%)	3 (16%)
Number of replies:	48	30	18

Percentages are of total number of replies in each column

Table 7.7 Loudness of tinnitus

Assessment	Numbers of children		
	Total	PHUs	Schools
Quiet	22 (54%)	10 (45%)	12 (67%)
Medium	13 (33%)	9 (41%)	4 (22%)
Very loud	5 (13%)	3 (14%)	2 (11%)
Number of replies:	40	22	18

Percentages are of total number of replies in each column

Table 7.8 Degrees of annoyance caused by tinnitus

		Numbers of children		
Annoyance	Grade	Total	PHUs	Schools
Not at all	0	20 (27%)	17 (30%)	3 (18%)
Slightly	1	22 (30%)	16 (28%)	6 (35%)
Sometimes	2	24 (32%)	18 (32%)	6 (35%)
Always	3	8 (11%)	6 (11%)	2 (12%)
Number of replies:		74	57	17

Percentages are of total number of replies in each column

Table 7.9 High Annoyance Children

Numbers of children with tinnitus	78
Children with high degree of annoyance:	
Total:	24 (31%)
of 59 children in PHUs	17 (29%)
of 19 children in schools for the deaf	7 (37%)

there were about 7000 children of secondary school age in PHUs and schools for the deaf in England and Wales, a crude extrapolation of these figures suggests a population of 1300 such children with annoying tinnitus.

Audiometry, hearing aids and tinnitus

Two important aspects of tinnitus in children are related to audiometry and hearing aids. We identified a small group of children (Graham & Butler 1984) in whom tinnitus made audiometry difficult. Many adults say that the more carefully they listen, the louder their tinnitus becomes: these children may have had a similar problem. The main difficulty, however, was that when audiometry was performed in the usual way, presenting loud tones first, these high-intensity sounds provoked or exacerbated the tinnitus. These children had been identified by their teacher (Brown 1981) as giving slow responses and inconsistent thresholds during routine audiometry.

We confirmed that they found it very hard to give reliable thresholds when pure tones were presented first loudly, then more quietly ('descending audiometry'). However when the tones were presented quietly, below threshold, and then with increasing loudness ('ascending audiometry'), these children gave much brisker responses and the thresholds obtained were confidently confirmed on retesting. Figures 7.1 and 7.2 show examples where the thresholds obtained by ascending audiometry were better than those previously shown by conventional testing. Figure 7.3 shows the opposite effect, produced by false positive responses. Normally, descending audiometry gives better thresholds than ascending; the usual exception in non-organic deafness. However any doubt about the accuracy of the new thresholds obtained by ascending audiometry in these children was dispelled by their increased confidence and faster reaction times. Further, the children whose audiograms are shown in Figures 7.1 and 7.3 had unilateral tinnitus (and bilateral deafness) and

138 TINNITUS

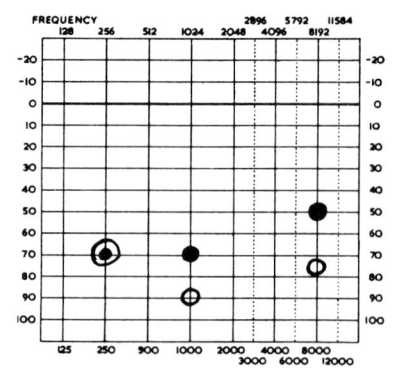

Fig. 7.1 Child of 12 with tinnitus provoked by audiometry. Open circles show thresholds obtained by conventional 'descending intensity' audiometry. Solid circles show better and more reliable thresholds obtained by 'ascending intensity' audiometry.

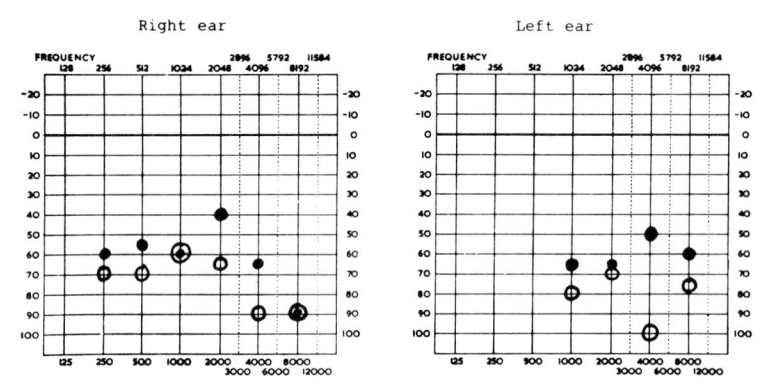

Fig. 7.2 Child of 13 with bilateral tinnitus provoked by audiometry. Notorious at school for unreliable audiograms. Open circles show responses obtained by conventional audiometry. Closed circles show responses using 'ascending intensity' audiometry.

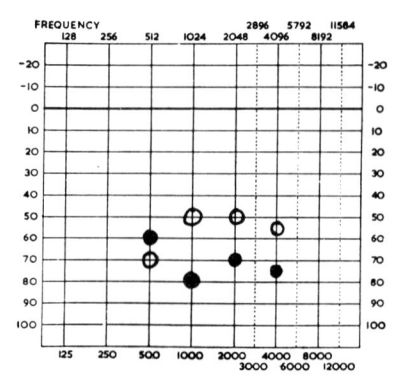

Fig. 7.3 Child of 15 with right-sided tinnitus matched with narrow-band noise at 7 kHz. Open circles show thresholds obtained by conventional audiometry, closed circles using 'ascending intensity' audiometry, which gave higher but much more consistent thresholds.

neither child had ever experienced any difficulty in performing audiometry with the ear that was not affected by tinnitus.

Tinnitus may be a complication of hearing-aid use; it may make a child reluctant to wear aids and it can explain why a certain aid or volume and tone adjustment is preferred or rejected for no obvious reason. This is demonstrated clearly in two children with unilateral tinnitus whose ears did not behave symmetrically. In one, the ear with tinnitus had a 'trough'-shaped audiogram curve with relatively good high-frequency hearing; the opposite ear had a sloping high-frequency loss. He wore two identical aids with powerful high-frequency responses and his tinnitus appeared in the ear with the 'trough' audiogram every morning if he put his aids on for as little as a minute then removed them. The second child appeared to have identical sloping, high-frequency hearing losses in both ears, but only the ear with tinnitus showed clear evidence of recruitment. It seemed inappropriate that both these children should be wearing pairs of identical hearing aids when their ears were far from identical in behaviour; in each case the ear with tinnitus needed an aid with some form of automatic volume control and a reduced high-frequency output.

PALATAL MYOCLONUS

In 1980 a children's book called 'Clicking Vicky' (Freud 1980) appeared about a small girl with palatal myoclonus. This symptom was described by Politzer (1878) and consists of irregular clicks associated with twitches in the muscles of the palate (MacKinon 1968), audible to an observer using a microphone in the external auditory meatus or a rubber tube placed in the patient's ear. Hazell (1984) reported the successful use of tinnitus masking in patients suffering from palatal myoclonus; two of the cases quoted (Hazell 1985) were children. A 13-year-old boy had myoclonus for five years; the symptom was controlled by unilateral masking which produced 30 minutes' residual inhibition. A 12-year-old's myoclonus, present for one year, was reduced and then abolished after using a masker for two months.

VENOUS HUMS

These are well recognised by cardiologists. The child hears a low-frequency hum, varying in intensity with respiration. This hum can usually be heard by placing a stethoscope on the child's neck. It is altered when the child holds his breath and usually abolished by gentle pressure over the internal jugular vein in the neck. The hum is ascribed to turbulence in the internal jugular vein: however, in some adults angiography has demonstrated arterio-venous fistulae in the intracranial circulation. It would be hard to justify angiography in a child with a venous hum and even harder to justify any form of operation, such as ligation of the internal jugular vein. Hums tend to become quieter as the child grows; if the hum is very troublesome masking can suppress it without, of course, producing residual inhibition.

MANAGEMENT OF A CHILD WITH TINNITUS

'It gets on my blooming nerves, please do something about it and quick'. Allowing for the cockney tendency for dramatic hyperbole this unsolicited remark from one of the children replying to a questionnaire suggests a considerable degree of annoyance. Statistics are not very helpful when you have to deal with an individual patient. I doubt if this child would be pleased to hear that the only 'something . . . quick' that I have done following his cry for help was to drop yet another paper into the ever-rolling stream of medical literature. The protocol described in Appendix 7.2 (Graham & Butler 1984) was designed to be used, in schools if necessary, with any standard portable audiometer, a portable acoustic impedance machine and a stethoscope. Tinnitus is not uniform in its aetiology, its behaviour or its effects. Clinical management relies on knowing as much as possible about the behaviour of the tinnitus in an individual child. Having found out as much as possible about the behaviour of a child's tinnitus the clinician may be able to offer help in various ways.

Hearing aids

As described above, tinnitus may be provoked by inappropriate hearing aids; changing the aid or its setting may help.

Audiometry

The most helpful thing for a child who finds audiometry difficult because of tinnitus may be to identify the reason for the problem and explain it to the teacher or the audiometrician. 'Ascending' audiometry seems to help children with this problem. In a few cases the tinnitus can be abolished for a few minutes by masking. During this period audiometry is much easier.

Masking

In 1984 (Butler & Graham 1984) we reported the findings in a small series of seven children fitted with maskers by my colleague Jonathan Hazell. He found that the benefit gained by masking was worthwhile. Three children had complete control of their tinnitus: in two there was residual inhibition and in one the tinnitus was completely abolished. The other four children said that masking, while not completely suppressing their tinnitus, produced an adequate degree of control.

General measures

From the degree of annoyance reported earlier in this chapter, tinnitus would be expected to produce changes in a child's behaviour and ability to concentrate. Since tinnitus in children is almost always intermittent it should be suspected in a deaf child whose behaviour is erratic for no obvious reason.

CONCLUSION

Tinnitus seems only recently to have been recognised as common in deaf children. Although it is seldom mentioned many children seem to find it annoying; it has been shown to have a clear effect on audiometry and hearing-aid use in some children and is likely to have less easily measurable effects on the behaviour of deaf children, both in and out of school.

Acknowledgements

The Ciba Foundation kindly gave me permission to use Tables 7.1–7.8. Jane Butler has given enthusiastic help and much thoughtful advice. Janet Brown has kindly provided a stream of deaf pupils and the facilities of her partial hearing unit in Chalk Farm. Pat Garrett patiently and expertly typed and retyped the manuscript.

REFERENCES

Alpers B J 1960 Vertiginous epilepsy. Laryngoscope 70: 631–637
Brown J 1981 Personal communication
Coles R R A 1984 Epidemiology of tinnitus; (2) demographic and clinical features. In: Proceedings of the Second International Tinnitus Seminar, New York, 1983. Journal of Laryngology and Otology Supplement 9: 195–202
Coles R R A, Davis A C, Haggard M P 1981 Epidemiology of tinnitus. In: Evered D, Lawrenson G (eds) Tinnitus. Ciba Foundation Symposium 85, Pitman, London, pp 16–34
Emmett J R 1981 In: Evered D, Lawrenson G (eds) Tinnitus. Ciba Foundation Symposium 85, Pitman, London, p 182
Freud C 1980 Clicking Vicky, Pelham Books, London
Glanville J D, Coles R A, Sullivan B M 1971 A family with high-tonal objective tinnitus. Journal of Laryngology and Otology 85: 1–10
Goodey R J 1981 In: Evered D, Lawrenson G (eds) Tinnitus. Ciba Foundation Symposium 85, Pitman, London, p 183
Graham J M 1981a Paediatric tinnitus. In: Proceedings of the First International Tinnitus Seminar, New York 1979. Journal of Laryngology and Otology. Supplement 4: 117–120
Graham J M 1981b Tinnitus in children with hearing loss. In: Evered D, Lawrenson G (eds) Tinnitus. Ciba Foundation Symposium 85, Pitman, London, pp 172–181
Graham J M, Butler J 1984 Tinnitus in children. In: Proceedings of the Second International Tinnitus Seminar, New York 1983. Journal of Laryngology and Otology. Supplement 9: 236–241
Hazell J W P 1981 Patterns of tinnitus. Medical audiologic findings. In: Proceedings of the First International Tinnitus Seminar, New York 1979. Journal of Laryngology and Otology. Supplement 4: 39–47
Hazell J W P 1984 Discussion on tinnitus masking. In: Proceedings of the Second International Tinnitus Seminar, New York 1983. Journal of Laryngology and Otology. Supplement 9: 253
Hazell J W P 1985 Personal communication
Illum P 1972 The Mondini type of cochlear malformation. A survey of the literature. Archives of Otolaryngology 96: 305–311
Kemp D T 1981 In: Evered D, Lawrenson G (eds) Tinnitus. Ciba Foundation Symposium 85: (Discussion). Pitman, London, p 184
MacKinnon D M 1968 Objective tinnitus due to palatal myoclonus. Journal of Laryngology and Otology 82: 369–374
Nodar R H 1972 Tinnitus aurium in school age children: a survey. Journal of Auditory Research 12: 133–135
Nodar R H, LeZak M H W 1984 Pediatric tinnitus (a thesis revisited). In: Proceedings of the Second International Tinnitus Seminar, New York 1983. Journal of Laryngology and Otology. Supplement 9: 234–235
Politzer A 1978 Palatal myoclonus. Lehrbuch der Ohrenheilkunde. Enke Verlag, Stuttgart
Reich G 1981 Personal communication
Snashall S E 1984 Vertigo in children. In: Dix M R, Hood J D (eds) Vertigo. Wiley, Chichester, pp 267–289

APPENDIX 7.1

Questions used in the survey of tinnitus among children of secondary-school age

Questions

1. Does the noise appear to come from your left ear/right ear/both ears?
2. Which ear do you wear your aid on: left/right/both?
3. Which is the noise most like: whistling/ringing/rushing?
4. Is the noise there all the time/only sometimes?
5. If the noise is there sometimes, is it when you are relaxed/tense? or if at any other regular time please state here:
6. When in a noisy place or using a hearing aid are the noises in your head reduced/no change/greater?
7. Is the noise like a pulse?
8. Does the noise worry you not at all/slightly/all the time?
9. Have you ever had ear infections or had to have an operation to take fluid away from the middle ear, grommets, etc?

Supplementary questions

10. If the noise is not there all the time, about how often do you get it?
    Every day/every week (about how many times a week?)/every month (about how many times a month?)/less often (how often?)
11. When you get the noise, how long does it usually last?
    Seconds/minutes (how many?)/hours (how many?)/days (how many?)
12. How loud is the noise?
13. When you hear the noise does it make your hearing worse?
14. Does it make it difficult for you to hear people's voices?
15. When you get the noise do you feel dizzy or have trouble with your balance?
16. When you get the noise do you notice anything else?

APPENDIX 7.2

Protocol for assessing tinnitus in hearing-impaired children

1. General details
    Age
    Sex
    Pure tone audiometry
    Better hearing ear
    Medical diagnosis if known
    Aids: side and type

2. Description of tinnitus
    Side
    Description
    Loudness
    Annoyance
    Provoking factors
    Frequency
    Duration

3. If tinnitus is not present at the time of examination there are various manoeuvres which may provoke it
    Aids turned off
    Aids removed
    Ear defenders (headphones)
    Lie down
    Exercise
    Shake head
    Exposure to sound

   In addition to these manoeuvres the child may suggest some further manoeuvre which may provoke the tinnitus.
   To a child who states that he develops tinnitus after exposure to loud noises we present pure tones at 250 Hz, 2 kHz and 9 kHz and white noise for 30 s in one or both ears at 100–110 dB.

4. If tinnitus cannot be provoked, then the child is given an appointment to come back on a different occasion

5. If the tinnitus is either present from the beginning of the consultation or can be provoked by one of the manoevres mentioned above, the following basic list of tests is presented.
    Otoscopy
    Listening for audible tinnitus using low impedance microphone and occuluded external auditory meatus
    Listening over neck with stethoscope for venous hum
    Change in subjective loudness of tinnitus with ears occluded and with ear defenders
    Frequency match using pure tones or narrow band noise
    Ascending audiometry
    Descending audiometry
    Pulsed audiometry
    Loudness discomfort levels
    White noise threshold and tinnitus masking level using white noise
    Residual inhibition after 60 seconds masking noise at 10 dB masking level
    Impedance measurement and stapedius reflex thresholds

Surgical management of the tinnitus patient

At present surgery has a relatively small place in the management of patients presenting with tinnitus. Sensorineural tinnitus originating in the cochlea or auditory tract would be regarded by some as 'tinnitus proper' and would certainly account for the vast majority of cases seen by any otologist or audiologist. Nevertheless any persistent noise generated in or around the head can be troublesome and may present to a tinnitus, audiology or otology clinic. In some cases sounds are being generated by, for instance, crepitus in the cervical spine, or temporomandibular joint. However much these entities may represent totally different and diverse pathologies, and are nothing to do with the ear, it is important to be aware of these conditions and to be able to institute correct investigation and management.

Patients with conductive deafness may often be helped by surgery, and it is important to be able to give a separate prognosis about the effects of such intervention on both hearing and tinnitus. Some patients with a sensorineural hearing loss and tinnitus, notably with Ménière's disease, perilymph fistula or acoustic neuroma, may also expect improvement of their tinnitus as a result of surgical management.

The majority of papers concerned with the effects of surgery on tinnitus are reports of auditory and vestibular nerve section and labyrinthectomy. Ninety percent of the cases presented are of Ménière's disease or acoustic neuroma. These are relatively rare conditions in the general population compared to the very high incidence of 'idiopathic sensorineural tinnitus'. These surgical studies should not be used to extrapolate what might happen if destructive procedures were employed more widely in idiopathic cases. In the majority of pure tinnitus cases the presence of useful hearing in the affected ear precludes any such therapeutic approach.

The surgical management of any ear condition should be influenced by the part that tinnitus plays in the patient's complaint. It should always be remembered that surgical failures may result in the most severe and troublesome tinnitus and where this occurs in a dead ear, it may even be extremely difficult to treat. On the other hand it may be necessary to operate on an ear in an effort to preserve residual hearing so that masking techniques may still be employed. Those centres who have enjoyed some success from masking techniques have changed their philosophy from one of advocating labyrinthectomy because a hearing-impaired ear has no speech discrimination, to one of conservation of residual hearing so that tinnitus may still be controlled by prosthetic management.

PULSATILE TINNITUS

Tinnitus which is pulsatile, usually in synchrony with the pulse, is the most prominent complaint in 12% of tinnitus sufferers. Right and left ears are equally affected. In a group of 200 patients pulsatile tinnitus was never described as 'in the head' (Hazell et al 1985). However, an audible bruit is present in only a small proportion of patients with pulsatile tinnitus (Tewfik 1984). There are many sources of vascular sound in and around the ear including transmitted pulsations from meningial vessels through a patent cochlear aqueduct, abnormal stria vascularis circulation, and arteriovenous malformations around the ear which may have special surgical significance. Pulsatile tinnitus occurs in Paget's disease (Gibson 1973).

Holgate et al (1977) have discussed the role of angiography in pulsatile tinnitus and have divided the different abnormalities into arteriovenous shunts, arterial shunts or anastomoses, and irregular lumens, from whom the following scheme is adapted.

a. Arteriovenous shunts

    Congenital arteriovenous malformations
    Acquired   — arteriovenous fistulae
                 — tumours: glomus jugulare
                             acoustic neuroma
                             meningioma
                             metastatic
    Paget's disease

b. Arterio-arterial shunts

    Congenital — primitive otic artery
                    — primitive hypoglossal artery
                    — persistant stapedial artery
    Acquired   — contralateral carotid occlusion

c. Venous hums

            — abnormal jugular bulb
            — intracranial hypertension

d. Other arterial bruits

            — carotid stenosis
            — vascular loops in the internal auditory meatus
            — transmission of cardiac murmurs

Venous hums

Several authors have described the presence of a pulsatile tinnitus with very characteristic properties. Pulse synchronous sounds are heard on one side only, and rotation of the head to the opposite side increases their loudness. They are reduced by rotation or flexion of the head to the affected side. Light pressure on the internal jugular vein, insufficient to occlude the carotid artery, abolishes the sound. This led to the description by Carey (1961) of a prosthetic device which lightly pressed on the jugular vein. The pulsation may usually be heard with a stethoscope placed over the neck or external auditory meatus. Ligation of the jugular vein in the neck has been suggested (Chandler 1983, Ward et al 1975, Rothstein et al 1985. George et al (1983) combined ligation of the jugular vein with a lateral sinus/jugular vein anastomosis. Meador and Swift (1984) describe five patients with a venous hum obliterated by light pressure on the jugular vein. In each case there was a raised intracranial pressure which could be detected by lumbar puncture. In their series the pressure ranged from 260 mm H_2O to 360 mm H_2O. Their cases included idiopathic communicating hydrocephalus, pseudo tumor cerebri and a primary brain tumour (cystic astroblastoma). Two cases were treated with subarachnoid peritoneal shunt with disappearance of tinnitus symptoms. They postulate that the mechanism in this case is due to a venous bruit resulting from turbulence created as blood flows from the hypertensive intracranial portion into the low pressure of the jugular bowl. The symptom is unilateral due to asymmetry of the jugular bulb. They demonstrate the importance of excluding raised intracranial pressure before contemplating jugular ligation.

Arteriovenous malformations

Arteriovenous malformations have been described by Arenberg & McCreary (1971), Vallis & Martin (1984) and Ward et al (1975). Ward et al (1975) point out that branches of the occipital artery and transverse sinus are commonly involved in arteriovenous malformations, as there are numerous interconnections between these vessels. Frequently there is no history of trauma. Branches of the internal carotid and vertebral artery may also produce fistulae. Less commonly there are vascular abnormalities in the middle fossa between the posterior branches of the middle meningial artery and greater petrosal sinus. Connection between the internal carotid artery and the cavernous sinus almost always follows severe head trauma (Boulet et al 1985). Arenberg & McCreary describe three cases of arteriovenous malformations between the terminal branches of the external carotid artery and the transverse sinus. Newton et al (1968) describe a detailed study of 17 dual arteriovenous malformations of the posterior fossa. In nine, venous drainage was primarily into the transverse sinus. Where pulsatile tinnitus is a troublesome feature, surgical removal of the lesion or ligation of its blood supply is often effective.

Harris et al (1979) described the management of 15 patients with severe pulsatile tinnitus. Selective angiography gave a positive diagnosis in 12 of the 15 cases revealing glomus jugulare tumour in 3, arterial malformations in 8 and stenosis of the carotid artery in one. Embolization using absorbable gelatin sponge was employed, cut into thin strips measuring $1 \times 1 \times 8$ mm. Contrast medium was injected immediately before and after each embolization following fluoroscopy to check the position of the catheter tip. The number of emboli required for occlusion of the feeding vessels varied from 1 to over 20. Embolization was performed once in six patients, twice in three and three times in two patients. A lasting satisfactory effect in terms of the pulsatile tinnitus was achieved in 75% of cases. Digital subtraction angiographic techniques may be helpful in identifying larger lesions (Carmody et al 1983) and Leveque et al (1979) have shown how routine tympanometry may identify and provide a record of abnormal vascular activity in the ear.

VASCULAR LOOPS IN THE INTERNAL AUDITORY CANAL

Anatomical studies have shown that the loop of the anterior inferior cerebellar artery not infrequently enters the internal auditory canal, producing compression on the eighth cranial nerve (Kudo & Ito 1984). In a series of 150 CT studies of the cerebellar pontine angle and internal auditory meatus, Appelbaum & Valvassori (1984) detected 10 patients with a prominent cascular loop in the IAM in close relationship to the eighth nerve. Eight of these patients had tinnitus and three had vertiginous episodes. Jannetta (1980) has reported on the results of surgical decompression of the eighth nerve for symptoms of tinnitus and vertigo in 38 patients. About two-thirds were improved by surgery, the remaining third being unchanged or becoming worse. In general the results for vertigo were better than those for tinnitus. Bertrand et al (1977) described a series of five patients with vascular loop compression: in three patients the symptoms were improved.

PATULOUS EUSTACHIAN TUBE

In this condition the patient often complains of a roaring sound in the ear. Interestingly, they may be unaware that this is synchronous with nasal respiration. There is also a feeling of fullness and paradoxical blocking of the ear and the patient's voice may produce reverberant effects within the ear, particularly to consonant sounds such as 'm' or 'n'. The symptoms often disappear on bending the head down between the knees (by producing venous engorgement of the tubal mucosa). There may have been a history of recent weight loss (resulting in loss of peritubal fat). On examination, the tympanic membrane often moves with nasal respiration and is usually easily visible, if not with an auriscope then with the added magnification afforded by the operating microscope (Schwartze, cited by Ogawara 1976). The posterior superior quadrant of the tympanic membrane is often thin and atrophic. Auscultation of the ear frequently reveals the amplified sound of nasal respiration and occasionally the distortion effects experienced by the patient on speaking. Epley (1981) described a small amplifier connecting the external meatus and the nasal vestibule which produces a feedback squeak indicating abnormal patency of the Eustachian tube in this syndrome.

Many different surgical techniques have been tried to reduce the lumen of the Eustachian tube and these are summarised by O'Connor & Shea (1981). They report seven cases treated by application of 20% silver nitrate to the Eustachian tube via the nasopharynx. All reported improvement in autophony, and only one had persistent serous otitis media after treatment. Pulec (1967) describes the use of an injection of

Teflon® into the Eustachian cushions of 26 patients with patulous Eustachian tubes. At a 3-year follow-up 19 patients reported complete relief of their symptoms following one injection of Teflon®. In resistant cases we have used the judicious application of monopolar diathermy using a fine ureteric diathermy probe, improving on a technique described by Halstead (1926). Stroud et al reported in 1974 on a technique which involved transposition of the tensor velipalatini, the muscle responsible for opening the Eustachian tube during the process of yawning and swallowing etc. Three patients obtained improvement of their symptoms.

THE ROLE OF THE INTRATYMPANIC MUSCLES

The function of the middle ear muscles has been variously described by Klochoff (1961), Anderson (1974) and Wiggers (1937). The importance of the generation of tinnitus lies in the possibility of surgical intervention. A very careful history must be taken to avoid missing these unusual presentations of tinnitus. So often patients so affected are labelled as having psychosomatic disturbance.

Idiopathic stapedial muscle spasm

In this condition the patient complains of a crackling or rustling noise in the ear in response to hearing certain sounds, generally loud sounds, and often of certain specific frequencies. Marchiando et al (1983) describe two patients in whom the symptom was abolished by section of the stapedius muscle. The condition has also been described in eight patients with associated facial nerve paralysis in whom the tinnitus occurred with eyelid blinking (Watanabe et al 1974). Again stapedial tenotomy relieved the symptom. We have confirmed this diagnosis in four patients. One patient had already undergone a tympanotomy for subluxation of the incudo stapedial joint and in this patient the rustling sound could be elicited not only by the application of loud tones above 70 dB SPL (sound pressure level), but also by touching the skin of the cheek, suggesting that the tensor tympani was also involved in mediating the response. Examination of the tympanic membrane under the highest power of the operating microscope revealed a very clear movement of the tympanic membrane in synchrony with the phenomenon, and in common with our other cases and those described in the literature a small compliance change could be detected on impedance audiometry when the sound stimulus was applied. Stapedius and tensor tympani tenotomy abolished the symptoms. It was supposed that the sound was produced by a form of crepitus coming from the ossicular chain or tympanic membrane. This was supported in another similar case where there was a very thin and mobile atrophic segment to the tympanic membrane in the pars flaccida. Surgical attention to this defect abolished the symptoms.

Myoclonus

Irregular clicking sounds in the ear associated with synchronous movements of the soft palate was first described by Politzer in 1862 (Gallet 1927). Although in the majority of cases the clicks are considered to be made by the mucous membrane of the Eustachian tube snapping together (MacKinnon 1968), there is also evidence that the intratympanic muscles may be involved in this process as well (Watanabe et al 1974). Lusk & Babin (1985) reported synkinetic contaction of the tensor tympani with the masseter muscle causing tinnitus. In sensorineural tinnitus an almost universal experience is that the amplitude of tinnitus increases on clenching the teeth. Corresponding increases in intra-tympanic muscle tone so caused could result in a decrease of middle-ear compliance and a tendency for mechanical or resonant activity in the cochlea to be reflected back into it from the stapedial footplate (Wilson & Sutton 1981). It is reasonable to suppose that increased tension in the pterygoid muscles which can occur in the temporomandibular joint syndrome may result in increased muscle tone in other muscles having the same innovation including the tensor tympani (Costen 1937, Arlen 1977, Gelb & Bernstein 1983). Klochoff (1981) describes an impedance fluctuation detectable on impedance audiometry in 76 cases with 'tensor tympani' syndrome. He postulates that a tonic tensor activity accounts for symptoms of fullness in the ear, tinnitus and dysacusis. Tension headache and vertigo (dizziness and dysequilibrium) were present in over 80% of cases. These patients were managed by reassurance and counselling; intratympanic muscles section had not been performed, although this could be contemplated in certain cases (Klochoff 1985).

SURGERY FOR DEAFNESS: THE EFFECTS ON TINNITUS

Conductive deafness

Tinnitus is a relatively uncommon presenting symptom in conductive deafness. Hazell et al (1985) in a study of 472 patients presenting with a primary complaint of tinnitus made a diagnosis of otitis in 6% and otosclerosis in 4%. (Noise-induced hearing loss and acoustic trauma accounted for 27% of cases and the diagnosis was not determined in 44%.) Reed in 1960 reported on 200 cases of tinnitus with a 3% incidence of middle ear or Eustachian tube disease, and 7.5% of otosclerosis. Some authors have commented on the low incidence of troublesome tinnitus in middle ear disease. In 1946 Lempert reported the effect of tympano-sympathectomy after several patients reported improvement of their tinnitus following radical mastoidectomy for chronic ear infection. Ten of the 15 patients were reported to have complete relief of their symptoms.

In the recent literature there are no reports of the prevalence of tinnitus in tympanic membrane perforation, or of the effects of myringoplasty. Sheehy & Anderson in 1980, reviewing 472 cases of myringoplasty, regretted that the questionnaire circulated to their patients omitted mention of pre- or post-operative tinnitus. They felt that tinnitus was not related to the size of the air/bone gap either before or after the operation. Nevertheless it is most surgeons' clinical experience that tinnitus often lessens following improvement of the conductive deafness. The mechanism of tinnitus generation in such cases is likely to be noise generated in the cochlea or auditory tract increased by the earplug effect of the conductive loss. Restoring a more normal conductive mechanism eliminates this effect and allows environmental masking to act on the cochlea. An improvement in hearing, even a complete closure of the air/bone gap, is not invariably associated with an improvement in tinnitus; indeed in some cases this may worsen, and all patients should be advised of this possibility prior to surgery.

In 1853 Toynbee described a prosthesis for covering the tympanic membrane perforation to improve the hearing. The pre-operative application of a small patch of sterile tissue paper (the patch test) can be most valuable in assessing the mechanical advantage that can be obtained by surgical closure of a perforation, and to establish the effect that surgical closure of the perforation may have both on the hearing and the tinnitus.

The effect of otosclerotic surgery on tinnitus is better documented. Glasgold and Altmann (1966) reported on the effects of stapes surgery on tinnitus in 190 cases. Different techniques were compared, including 34 cases who had stapes mobilisations. There was no significant difference between the techniques although among those patients who received fat wire prostheses (34 cases) there were no cases of tinnitus becoming louder post-operatively. Overall pre-operative tinnitus was present in 78.9%. No mention was made of the severity of the tinnitus pre-operatively. In most patients presenting with otosclerosis the hearing loss is more troublesome than the tinnitus. In those cases in which the post-operative air/bone closure was better than 15 dB for all frequencies, and in whom a stapedectomy had been performed, 31% had experienced disappearance of their tinnitus, in 33% it had decreased, in 23% it remained the same and in 3% it became louder. Causse et al (1983) report that only low and medium tone tinnitus usually disappear after stapedectomy. They suggest that tinnitus between 250 Hz and 1 kHz may be due to ossicular impedance changes or to high pressure of the labyrinthine fluids. Tinnitus (of otosclerosis) around 2 kHz they consider to be of enzymatic origin, which may be helped by sodium fluoride treatment. Bretlau et al (1985) report no significant improvement in otosclerotic tinnitus following fluoride therapy.

Sensorineural deafness

Although tinnitus is one of the triad of symptoms in Ménière's disease it is not often the most troublesome, except in 'burnt-out cases' where the devastating effects of paroxysmal vertigo and vomiting have ceased. Vernon et al (1981) report that in over 1200 patients presenting with the primary complaint of tinnitus, only 15 were diagnosed as having Ménière's disease. Hazell et al (1985) reported a 6% incidence in their study. The tinnitus is often low-pitched (Douek & Reid 1968) and this may be of diagnostic significance. Savary & Charissoux (1984) report the results of 218 operations on the endolymphatic sac for Ménière's disease. At 12 months after surgery tinnitus was eliminated in 34%, diminished in 39% and unchanged for 27%. Certainly the effects of endolymphatic sac surgery are better for the elimination of vertigo than for the improvement of tinnitus.

Perilymph fistula was first proposed as a cause of sudden hearing loss by Blair Simmons (1968). Goodhill et al in 1973 described labyrinthine window rupture and its repair at tympanotomy. Flood et al (1985) reported on 15 cases of labyrinthine window rupture repaired at tympanotomy and also described an audiometric test which shows changes in hearing with position in the presence of a perilymph leak. Improvement in hearing was obtained in only four cases and the effect on pre-operative tinnitus was not recorded. Experience suggests that although the tinnitus associated with perilymph fistula is more often than not unhelped by surgical closure of the leak, possibly because of irreversible damage to neural structures in the cochlea, this may well prevent further deterioration of hearing which could be important in the implementation of a programme of masking. Douek (1975) reported 27 cases of post-stapedectomy fistula in which 10 developed tinnitus. It was very severe in those who had profound hearing loss and was roaring in nature. The onset of the tinnitus was up to 6 years following the original stapedectomy operation. No details are available on the tinnitus following closure of the fistula but it was observed that it did not improve much, particularly if the pre-operative tinnitus had been severe.

DESTRUCTIVE SURGICAL PROCEDURES ON THE EAR: THE EFFECT ON TINNITUS

In cases of Ménière's disease where there is judged to be no useful hearing in the ear a membranous or bony labyrinthectomy may be performed with the primary aim of destroying the remaining vestibular function in the affected ear. Although this is an effective means of controlling vertigo, the most troublesome symptom in Ménière's disease, the effect on the tinnitus is more variable, and in addition any residual hearing which might be reached by a tinnitus masker is destroyed. Vernon et al (1980) note that in Ménière's disease the tinnitus can usually be easily masked regardless of the masking sounds. Our experience confirms this, and masking can be valuable even in those cases where there is quite a severe hearing loss. In those patients therefore, in whom the tinnitus is a troublesome feature, careful thought should be given to destructive surgery before the possibilities of medical treatment and surgery on the endolymphatic sac have been exhausted. Pedersen & Sorensen (1970) describe the results in 27 patients who reported tinnitus prior to operation. In 12 the tinnitus had ceased or diminished, but in 15 it was described as unchanged or aggravated.

Translabyrinthine section of the eighth nerve is commonly performed for severe Ménière's disease with little residual hearing. House and Brackmann (1981) report on 68 patients who had nerve section, usually of the vestibular nerve, but in some cases also the cochlear nerve. While only one patient admitted that the tinnitus had disappeared completely, 43% felt it was better but in 28% it had become worse. In 27% the tinnitus was uchanged. Pulec (1984) described the results in 93 patients with tinnitus in whom he performed translabyrinthine section of the cochlear nerve and both superior and inferior vestibular nerves. Of this series, 52 cases had Ménière's disease, 15 chronic otitis media, 9 post-stapedectomy, 9 trauma and 8 miscellaneous. Sixty-two patients received complete relief of their tinnitus and an improvement was obtained in 26. Only 5 patients obtained no improvement. However, Dandy (1941), describing his experience with tinnitus in 401 patients following acoustic nerve section for Ménière's disease, was less enthusiastic. He felt that 50% of the patients had an improvement in their tinnitus but that if the tinnitus persists it may not be improved. Of a series of 31 patients reported in Glasscock et al (1980), 72% felt that there was an improvement in their tinnitus. In surgery for acoustic neuroma the approach in most cases involves the removal of the bony labyrinth together with a section of the cochlear nerve, although occasionally some cochlea nerve function may be retained. House & Brackmann (1981) reviewed 500 consecutive patients who had acoustic neurectomy: 83% had tinnitus before surgery but only 11% said that it was their first symptom. Post-operatively, 40% of the patients felt their tinnitus was better, 50% said it was worse and only 10% found it to be the same as before.

Because of the good results with vestibular neurectomy in relieving the tinnitus of Ménière's disease, and because of the unreliable effects of cochlear nerve section, Fisch (1970) has excised the main trunk of the vestibular nerve in four patients with untreatable tinnitus. Three of them were relieved of their symptoms in the short term; two patients who had selective cochlear nerve section for severe tinnitus were unchanged. Glasscock et al (1984) confirmed the beneficial effect of total vestibular neurectomy on tinnitus in Ménière's disease, 61% reporting improvement.

Jackson (1985) agreed that the results of eighth nerve section for abolishing tinnitus were disappointing. He compared the effects of a bolus intravenous injection of lidocaine to the results of cochlear nerve section in seven patients. Although two patients whose tinnitus was not abolished by lidocaine improved on nerve section, there were no instances where a good response from the lidocaine test was followed by a poor operative result.

The results of destructive surgery are unpredictable, to say the least, as far as post-operative tinnitus is concerned. Even in a patient with no cochlear function, section of the cochlear nerve will preclude any possibility of electrical suppression of tinnitus via a cochlear implant (Ch. 6) (Fraysse & Lazorthes 1983). So far the available data relates largely to patients with Ménière's disease and acoustic neuroma in whom surgery was indicated for other reasons than tinnitus. The effects of ablative surgery in significant numbers of patients where tinnitus is the presenting symptom are unknown.

Acknowledgement

I am deeply grateful to Pat Garrett for taking this chapter through its many drafts, and for preparing the manuscript in its final form.

REFERENCES

Anderson D S 1974 The intratympanic muscles. Sci. Found. Otol. 257–259

Appelbaum F L, Valvassori G E 1984 Auditory and vestibular system findings in patients with vascular loops in the internal auditory canal. Annals of Otology Rhinology and Laryngology 93 (Supplement 112): 63–70

Arenberg I K, McCreary H S 1971 Objective tinnitus aurium and dural arterio-venous malformations of the posterior fossa. Annals of Otology Rhinology and Laryngology 80: 111–120

Arlen H 1977 The otomandibular syndrome. In: Clinical management of head, neck and TMJ pain and dysfunction. Gelb H (ed). Saunders, Philadelphia. pp 181–194

Bertrand R A, Molina P, Hardy J 1977 Vestibular syndrome and vascular anomaly in the cerebello-pontine angle. Acta Otolaryngologica 83: 187–194

Blair Simmons F 1968 Theory of membrane breaks in sudden hearing loss. Archives of Otolaryngology 88: 41–48

Boutet J J, Legent F, Beauvillain C, Duguet V, Galiba J 1985 Pulsatile tinnitus caused by preauricular vascular lesions of traumatic origin. Annales d'Otolarngologie et Chirurgie Cervico faciale 102: 251–253

Bretlau P, Causse J, Causse J B, Hansen H J, Johnsen N J, Salomon G 1985 Otospongiosis and sodium fluoride. A blind experimental and clinical evaluation of the effect of sodium fluoride treatment in patients with otospongiosis. Annals of Otology Rhinology and Laryngology 94: 103–107

Carey F H 1961 Symptomatic venous hum. New England Journal of Medicine 264: 869–870

Carmody R F, Seeger J F, Horsley W W, Smith J R, Miller R W 1983 Digital subtraction angiography of glomus tympanicum and jugulare tumours. American Journal of Neuroradiology 4: 263–265

Causse J B, Causse J R, Wiet R J, Yoo T J 1983 Complications of stapedectomies. American Journal of Otology 4: 275–280

Chandler J R 1983 Diagnosis and cure of venous hum tinnitus. Laryngoscope 93: 892–895

Costen J B 1937 Summary of neuralgias and ear symptoms associated with mandibular joint. Mississippi Doctor 15: 33

Dandy W E 1941 Surgical treatment of Ménière's disease. Surgery Gynecology and Obstetrics 72: 421–425

Douek E 1975 Perilymph fistula. Journal of Laryngology 89: 123–130

Douek E, Reid J 1968 The diagnostic value of tinnitus pitch. Journal of Laryngology 82: 1039–1042

Epley J M 1981 Electronic probe for eustachian tube patency and objective tinnitus. Otolaryngology and Head and Neck Surgery 89: 854–855

Fisch U 1970 Transtemporal surgery of the internal auditory canal. Advances in Otology, Rhinology and Laryngology 17: 203–240

Flood L M, Fraser J G, Hazell J W P, Rothera M P 1985 Perilymph fistula. Four-year experience with a new audiometric test. Journal of Laryngology 99: 671–676

Fraysse B, Lazorthes Y 1983 Implantation chronique d'electrode au niveau de la fenêtre ronde dans le traitement des bourdonnements. Journal Francais d'Oto-Rhino-Laryngologie 32: 307–310

Gallet J 1927 Le nystagmus du voile. Thesis, University of Paris

Gelb H, Bernstein I 1983 Comparison of three different populations with temporomandibular joint pain-dysfunction syndrome. Dental Clinics of North America 27: 495–503

George B, Reizine D, Laurian C, Riche M C, Merland J J 1983 Tinnitus of venous origin. Surgical treatment by the ligation of the jugular vein and lateral sinus jugular vein anastomosis. Journal of Neuroradiology 10: 23–30

Gibson R 1973 Tinnitus in Paget's disease with external carotid ligation. Journal of Laryngology 87: 299–301

Glasgold A, Altmann F 1966 The effect of stapes surgery on tinnitus in otosclerosis. Laryngoscope 76: 1524–1532

Glasscock M E, Davis W E, Hughes G B, Jackson C G 1980 Labyrinthectomy versus middle fossa vestibular nerve section in Ménière's disease. A critical evaluation of relief of vertigo. Annals of Otology Rhinology and Laryngology 89: 318–324

Glasscock M E, Kveton J F, Christiansen S G 1984 Middle fossa vestibular neurectomy: an update. Otolaryngology and Head and Neck Surgery 92: 216–220

Halstead T H 1926 Pathology and surgery of the eustachian tube. Archives of Otolaryngology 4: 189–195

Harris S, Brismar J, Cronqvist S 1979 Pulsatile tinnitus and therapeutic embolization. Acta Otolaryngologica 88: 220–226

Hazell J W P, Wood S M, Cooper H R et al 1985 A clinical study of tinnitus maskers. British Journal of Audiology 19: 65–146

Holgate R C, Wortzman G, Noyek A M, Mekerewicz L, Coates R M 1977 Pulsatile tinnitus: the role of angiography. Journal of Otolaryngology (Supplement) 6: 49–62

House J W, Brackmann D E 1981 Tinnitus: surgical treatment. In: Evered D, Lawrenson G (eds) Tinnitus. Ciba Foundation Symposium 85. Pitman, London, pp 204–216

Jackson P 1985 A comparison of the effects of eighth nerve section with lodocaine on tinnitus. Journal of Laryngology 99: 663–666

Jannetta P J 1980 Neurovascular compression in cranial nerve and systemic disease. Annals of Surgery 192: 518–524

Klochoff I 1961 Middle ear muscle reflexes in man. Acta Otolaryngologica Supplement 164

Klochoff I 1981 Impedance fluctuation and a 'tensor tympani' syndrome. In: Proceedings of 4th International Symposium on Acoustic Impedance Measurements. Penha and Pizarro (eds) Universidade Nova de Lisboa, Lisbon, pp 69–76

Klochoff I 1985 Personal communication

Kudo T, Ito K 1984 Microvascular decompression of the eighth cranial nerve for disabling tinnitus without vertigo: a case report. Neurosurgery 14: 338–340

Lempert J 1946 Tympanosympathectomy: surgical technique for the relief of tinnitus aurium. Archives of Otolaryngology 43: 199–212

Leveque H, Bialostozky F, Blanchard C L, Suter C M 1979 Tympanometry in the evaluation of vascular lesions of the middle ear and tinnitus of vascular origin. Laryngoscope 89: 1197–1218

Lusk R, Babin R 1985 Tensor tympani and masseter muscle synkinesis. Otolaryngology and Head and Neck Surgery 93: 555–558

MacKinnon D M 1968 Objective tinnitus due to palatal myoclonus. Journal of Laryngology 82: 369–374

Marchiando A, Per-Lee J H, Jackson R T 1983 Tinnitus due to Idiopathic Stapedial Muscle Spasm. Ear Nose and Throat Journal 62: 8–13

Meador K J, Swift T R 1984 Tinnitus from intracranial hypertension. Neurology 34: 1258–1261

Nelson J R 1968 Long-term effects of acoustic neuroma surgery. Archives of Otolaryngology 88: 675–686

Newton T H, Weidner W, Grietz T 1968 Dural arteriovenous malformation in the posterior fossa Radiology 90: 27–35

O'Connor A F, Shea J J 1981 Autophony and the patulous eustachian tube. Laryngoscope 91: 1427–1435

Ogawara S et al 1976 Patulous eustachian tube. A new treatment with infusion of absorbable gelatine sponge solution. Archives of Otolaryngology 102: 276–280

Pedersen C B, Sorensen H 1970 Clinical effects of labyrinthectomy. Archives of Otolaryngology 92: 307–310

Pulec J L 1967 Abnormally patent eustachian tubes: treatment with injection of poly-tetrafluoroethylene (teflon) paste. Laryngoscope 77: 1543–1554

Pulec J L 1984 Tinnitus: surgical therapy. American Journal of Otology 5: 479–480

Reed G F 1960 An audiometric study of 200 cases of subjective tinnitus. Archives of Otolaryngology 71: 84–94

Rothstein J, Hilger P A, Boies L R Jr 1985 Venous hum as the cause of reversible factitious sensorineural hearing loss. Annals of Otology 94: 267–268

Savary P, Charissoux G 1984 Surgical opening of the endolymphatic sac in Ménière's disease–our experience from 1962-80. Journal of Otolaryngology 13: 73–75

Sheehy J L, Anderson R G 1980 Myringoplasty. A review of 472 cases. Annals of Otology 89: 331–334

Stroud M H, Spector G J, Maisel R H 1974 Patulous estachian tube syndrome. Preliminary report of the use of the tensor veli palatini transposition procedure. Archives of Otolaryngology 99: 419–421

Tewfik S 1974 Phonocephalography. An objective diagnosis of tinnitus. Journal of Laryngology 88: 869–875

Toynbee J 1853 On the use of an artificial membrana tympani in cases of deafness dependent on perforation or destruction of the natural organ. Churchill, London

Vallis R C, Martin F W 1984 Extracranial arteriovenous malformation presenting as objective tinnitus. Journal of Laryngology 98: 1139–1142

Vernon J, Johnson R, Schleuning A 1980 The characteristics and natural history of tinnitus in Ménière's disease. Otolarynologic Clinics of North America 13: 611–619

Ward P H, Babin R, Calcaterra T C, Konrad H R 1975 Operative treatment of surgical lesions with objective tinnitus. Annals of Otology, Rhinology, Laryngology 84: 473–482

Watanabe I U, Kumagami H, Tsuda Y 1974 Tinnitus due to abnormal contraction of stapedial muscle. Otology Rhinology and Laryngology 36: 217–226

Wiggers H C 1937 The function of the intra-aural muscles. American Journal of Physiology 120: 771–780

Wilson J P, Sutton G 1981 Acoustic correlates of tonal tinnitus. In: Evered D, Lawrenson G (eds) Tinnitus. Ciba Foundation Symposium 85, Pitman, London, pp 82–107

9

R. S. Hallam

Psychological approaches to the evaluation and management of tinnitus distress

TINNITUS COMPLAINT: RELATIONSHIP TO PATHOPHYSIOLOGICAL FACTORS, REAL OR IMAGINED

The psychology of tinnitus can be taken back to the point at which an individual first notices an incongruous sound and attempts to understand its significance. The term 'incongruous' seems appropriate here because for some individuals, persistent noises which have no external source are regarded as normal. This is true of persons who, since childhood, have always heard noises and only later discover that this is not a phenomenon common to everyone. For them tinnitus noises are congruous with their general perceptions of the world until they discover the 'disorder'.

It is not known whether psychological factors are implicated in the underlying pathophysiology of this disorder. However, this is not claimed to be a frequent occurrence. Cases where the tinnitus is said to have been brought on by psychological factors or by watching a TV programme about it can be explained by arguing that the subject's attention was drawn to a previously unnoticed sensation. For the purposes of this chapter I shall not regard tinnitus as a psychogenic disorder. Having said this, there are strong grounds for believing that psychological factors play an important role in the processes of noticing, interpreting, reporting, worrying and complaining about incongruous sounds which, to an observer, and usually to the subject, appear to have no external origin. The management of the tinnitus patient can usefully draw upon these psychological considerations and therapy itself might be directed at psychological processes in order to bring about a significant alleviation of suffering. It is worth noting that the simple notion that tinnitus distress can be directly related to the loudness of noises is inadequate (see below).

From a psychological standpoint, it probably matters little how the noises have been caused, although different aetiologies may produce characteristic types of tinnitus noise with concomitant variation in the type and level of complaint. For example, some forms of clicking tinnitus are under voluntary control and these noises are less likely to be distressing.

From the patient's viewpoint, how he or she interprets the cause of the tinnitus is probably of far-reaching significance, and one of the first aims of the physician is to correct any unwarranted fears about malignant causes of the phenomenon. This reassurance may be sufficient to prevent further annoyance from the tinnitus.

Although it is natural that tinnitus sufferers should attribute the cause of the noise to a disorder of the body and seek medical help, it should be noted that this attribution is the outcome of an interpretive process. On first noticing an incongruous sound, many tinnitus sufferers describe going through a process of checking likely sources such as a faulty electrical switch. Within minutes, hours or sometimes weeks, it is realised that the noises must be 'in the head'. However, there is a group of people who remain convinced that the noises have an external acoustic source and they often complain to environmental health officers or any other body they consider responsible, such as the Gas Board (Walford 1979). These are not individuals who would normally be classified as 'deluded' or 'psychotic' although their beliefs may be very stubbornly held. They may become a considerable nuisance to various authorities even though their complaints have been seriously investigated by noise experts. It is not known why some tinnitus sufferers make an external causal attribution although the noises they complain of tend to be of low pitch, and low-pitched noises are normally more difficult to localise in space. These patients rarely seek medical help for their 'tinnitus'.

Tinnitus: a medical, psychological or psychiatric problem?

In a proportion of tinnitus sufferers it may be doubted whether there is underlying aural pathology at all. The body is not, intrinsically, a silent place and so some 'tuning-in' to normal body signals may occur. The normality of the tinnitus phenomenon is indicated by the fact that from about 20% (at age 20 years) to about 40% (at age 60 years) of the general population have experienced tinnitus at one time or other (Hinchcliffe 1961). Coles and his colleagues (1981) have confirmed this prevalence. Otologically normal individuals apparently hear whistles, rings, buzzes, etc when they are placed in extremely quiet environments (Heller & Bergmann 1953). This raises the question as to whether some people who report noises in the absence of any detectable pathology are simply paying attention to ubiquitous body signals of no general significance. This tendency might be associated with attention to a variety of other bodily sensations, a characteristic of individuals sometimes referred to as 'hypochondriacal' or 'somatising'. Reich & Johnson (1984) found that their most disturbed group of tinnitus patients, according to MMPI (Minnesota Multiphasic Personality Inventory) scales, was the group with tinnitus and no hearing loss. This might imply that complaint about tinnitus in the absence of signs of ear pathology is related to general psychological characteristics of the kind indicated.

However, it would be unprofitable to classify tinnitus patients on the basis of an assumed underlying organic basis into those with a 'medical' and those with a 'psychiatric' problem. There are no grounds for asserting that tinnitus which is indubitably associated with medical disorders will necessarily constitute a distressing symptom or that tinnitus which probably has no pathological basis necessarily indicates the presence of a psychiatric disorder. In any event, in our own work we have not found it useful to classify patients as organic or non-organic, medical or psychiatric. Moreover, even severe distress is not always indicative of the need for psychological therapy especially when the distress derives from misinformation or general mismanagement.

Given that there are so many potential causes of tinnitus, including the effect of commonly prescribed drugs, it seems wise to emphasise to the patient that the ear can be damaged in slight (and many) ways (which is not to say that tinnitus is an insignificant source of distress). Even when psychological problems are clearly present the validity of tinnitus as a sensory experience should be supported. The genuine nature of the tinnitus is indicated when consistent pitch matches can be produced, as is usually the case. Granted that the complaint is considered 'genuine', it can still be pointed out to the patient that the distress which it occasions is largely a function of other factors such as ambient noise levels, competing activities, beliefs regarding the noise and methods of coping. The classification and management of tinnitus complaints is a topic to which I shall return.

Noticing noises is likely to depend on a variety of environmental, psychological, and hearing factors, as well as features intrinsic to the noise itself (see below). The question whether there are typical 'tinnitus personality structures', i.e. whether certain types of person notice and complain about tinnitus (House 1981), has also been considered. McFadden (1982) notes that studies of the personalities of tinnitus patients have not been designed to reveal the separate influence of personality as cause, and personality as effect, of tinnitus. He argues (McFadden 1982 p 56) that simple logic indicates that tinnitus can be a symptom of various physiological anomalies of the auditory and other systems and that these conditions probably strike people of all personality types indiscriminately. Personality factors are, of course, likely to influence the level of complaint, possibly interacting with concomitant environmental stressors. As McFadden rightly states, a person may come to focus on tinnitus as an obvious symptom, and a 'cause' of all of his or her problems. He goes on to say that untangling the web of interactions between physiological and psychological factors (including stress and labelling tendencies) might be either too time-consuming or beyond the training of the typical hearing professional. Therefore the latter is often left in the position of deciding between psychotherapy (which the patient may resist as being inappropriate) and simple remedies such as 'slowing down' and 'learning to relax'.

What is clearly called for is a greater understanding of tinnitus complaint behaviour itself. This should eventually lead to the development of a pragmatic model for tinnitus management in which the medical, psychological and psychiatric contributions are clearly delineated. Some preliminary steps in this direction have been taken by Stephens (1984). At the pole of least complaint, the tinnitus might be envisaged as merely an incongruous noise which is quickly dismissed when the patient receives whatever medical diagnosis or treatment is appropriate and has this explained. At levels of greater complaint, counselling aimed specifically at dealing with the person's reaction to the noises and ways of managing them may be called for. In yet more complex cases, complaint about tinnitus may be considered as a calling card to obtain help for more severe psychological problems such as depressed mood, anxiety problems and phobias. Rarely, auditory hallucinations are detected, which are part of a more severe psychological disturbance.

There is no reason to suppose that tinnitus can be neatly classified as primarily a medical, psychological, or psychiatric problem. Indeed, rarely in medicine or psychology are classifications mutually exclusive. Consequently treatment can be offered from different quarters at the same time. What is clear is that tinnitus is an extremely common problem. It is both unnecessary and unrealistic to regard tinnitus distress as always requiring highly skilled or specialised therapeutic help. It is reasonable to expect that some short and simple methods of counselling could be developed which would significantly alleviate the distress of the great majority of sufferers. Tinnitus maskers may have an important contribution to make in a relatively straightforward approach to tinnitus management (see Ch. 5). However, the extent to which masking operates acoustically or through the counselling and reassurance that accompanies the medical attention is, as yet, uncertain (Stephens & Corcoran 1986).

A PSYCHOLOGICAL MODEL OF TINNITUS TOLERANCE

Assuming that it cannot be eliminated by acceptable means and that it is essentially benign, and taking a rational view of the matter, tinnitus could be regarded as an essentially irrelevant auditory signal. The phenomenon of attending to repetitive and irrelevant stimuli has been well studied by physiologists and psychologists in terms of the processes of orientation, attention, and habituation. A model of tinnitus tolerance drawing upon the literature has been described elsewhere (Hallam et al 1984). It is suggested that tinnitus can be likened to any other auditory stimulus to which a person may or may not attend. Attention to the noises is assumed to bring about distress either because it is associated with the attribution of some threatening state of affairs (e.g. the presence of a tumour) or because the act of attending interferes with activities more in tune with the needs of the moment (e.g. listening to a conversation, or getting to sleep). It is also suggested that habituation to tinnitus noises (and therefore tolerance) is the normal response, even though this process may take weeks, months or sometimes years. Suffering and complaint is therefore the exception and needs to be explained as a failure of habituation. At least six classes of variable should be considered as influencing the process of attending, which in turn is related to complaint. These variables can be subdivided into sensory, perceptual and individual factors (see Fig. 9.1). So the habituation model of tolerance takes into account:

1. The characteristics of the stimulus, e.g. intensity and quality; if continuous, the variability; if intermittent, the frequency and pattern of occurrence. It is assumed that noises which are more salient for any reason and also variable and irregular will require a longer period of habituation.
2. Environmental conditions, e.g. the relative intensity of other stimuli and the competing demands on attention. Relative intensity will depend on hearing level as well as ambient sound levels. For some individuals masking by natural sounds will occur. Different activities will be associated with different attentional demands and levels of attention. Performance on some tasks appears to diminish attention to the noises.
3. The 'meaning' or significance of the stimulus. It is assumed that the more meaningful a stimulus, the more attention it will receive.

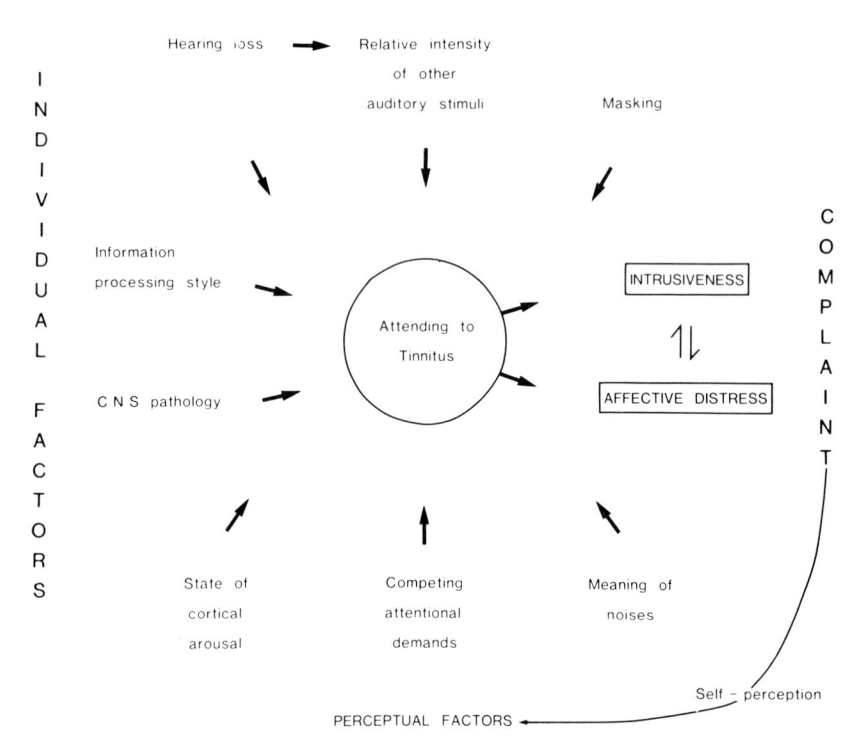

Fig. 9.1 Hypothetical model of tinnitus tolerance

4. Central state characteristics such as the level of cortical arousal. With increasing levels of cortical arousal, it is assumed that attention will become more highly focused and that habituation will be delayed.
5. General characteristics of the perceiver such as the style of information processing and general distractibility.
6. Organic pathology in the central nervous system affecting the neural pathways involved in attention and habituation.

This is not the place to expand on this general model but the variables considered above draw attention to many possible lines of enquiry (see Hallam et al 1984). The general model of tinnitus tolerance is supported by a variety of evidence. First, it is clear from epidemiological studies (Hinchcliffe 1961, Coles et al 1981) that many more people report tinnitus than are actually distressed or handicapped. Secondly, the model is broadly consistent with what tinnitus patients report as their sequence of reactions to tinnitus, i.e. the development of tolerance (see Hallam et al 1984). Thirdly, a survey of tinnitus club members indicated that the number of complaints tends to decline the longer the tinnitus had been present (Tyler & Baker 1983). Fourthly, the ratio of 'tinnitus as a main complaint' to 'tinnitus merely reported' declines as a function of the number of years that have elapsed since tinnitus was first noticed, i.e. the complaining group are more likely to be composed of cases of recent onset (Hallam et al 1984).

The kinds of clinical observation that are consistent with the model include patients' accounts that tinnitus only became a problem with a change of environment and activity level (e.g. retiring to a 'quiet place in the country'), that the onset of tinnitus followed soon after receiving information about it through the media, and so on. It may be suspected that tinnitus is often 'present' but unnoticed until other factors draw attention to it (for example, conducting research on the subject!)

COMPLAINT IN RELATION TO AUDIOMETRIC AND SENSORY FEATURES OF TINNITUS

It is often assumed, though not explicitly stated, that tinnitus distress is unidimensional and a function of the 'loudness' of the tinnitus. According to the habituation model of tolerance outlined above, it might be expected that a variety of features of the tinnitus, and of the subject, could combine to produce 'distress' and that this is unlikely to be unidimensional or merely a function of 'loudness'. Research conducted by the author and his colleagues supports these assumptions. The question of dimensionality is really the following: do complaints about tinnitus tend to form a single correlated cluster or do they form separate clusters which are statistically independent of each other? Having answered this question, it is then meaningful to go on to ask whether the dimension(s) of tinnitus complaint are associated with other features of tinnitus noises such as their quality, their pitch and their 'intensity'. Features of tinnitus sensations will be considered first.

Sensory aspects of tinnitus

A tinnitus noise may be intermittent, continuous, able to be matched to a spectrally simple or complex sound, seem to emanate from one or both ears, or the head, be pulsatile or hissing, and so on. Although attempts have been made to measure the quality of tinnitus (see McFadden 1982) there has been little success in relating qualitative features to aspects of complaint (Reed 1960; Hazell 1981a). It would appear that even intermittent tinnitus, if sufficiently frequent, can be as troublesome as continuous tinnitus (Office of Population Censuses and Surveys 1983).

An important feature of tinnitus is how readily it can be masked by external sounds (i.e. the level and frequencies of sound at which masking occurs). This feature is clearly relevant to the provision of maskers (discussed in Ch. 5) and it may also be relevant to complaint. Not all tinnitus is maskable (Mitchell 1983) but some tinnitus is masked by very low levels of sound. McFadden (1982, p 37) discusses these issues and also comments on the findings of Penner et al (1981) that the sound level required to continuously mask a tinnitus shows a rapid increase over 10 to 15 minutes before flattening off. (This is unlike the physical masking of one external sound by another). McFadden suggests that this may be one explanation why tinnitus continues to annoy even in relatively high-noise backgrounds.

The level of sound required to just mask tinnitus (minimal masking level MML) is often determined in tinnitus assessment procedures, especially when the provision of a masker is considered. This is an indirect measure of tinnitus 'intensity' although loudness-matching (Fowler 1936) is more commonly employed for this purpose. Despite numerous technical problems with the loudness-matching procedure (McFadden 1982 p 42) this remains a useful tool for investigating the hypothesis that tinnitus complaint (including self-reported loudness) is related to tinnitus loudness or 'intensity'.

Traditional loudness-match procedures which involve matching tinnitus to a sound delivered to the contralateral ear have tended to produce levels considered to be low given the amount of distress that is often expressed. These values are usually less than 15 dB sensation level (SL) (Reed 1960, Goodwin & Johnson 1980).

What these levels mean to the subject can be judged to some extent by comparing the loudness match to the values corresponding to the subject's judgements of his or her most comfortable loudness level — MCLL — as well as to the sound levels corresponding to half and twice the most comfortable loudness (Hinchcliffe & Chambers 1983). Individual loudness functions can be derived from these values, and the tinnitus loudness match expressed in personal loudness units (PLUs). It would appear that, on average, tinnitus is matched to a sound level which is considerably lower than the level corresponding to the subject's MCLL. In other words, in only a minority of distressed tinnitus patients does the tinnitus approach itensities that could be described as aversive (Hallam et al 1986). This finding is consistent with the view that tinnitus distress is not primarily determined by tinnitus 'intensity' (loudness) although, for some individuals at least, tinnitus is certainly *loud* and complaint is often observed to vary with variation in self-reported loudness.

What, first of all, is the evidence that loudness-match values correlate with loudness measured on a self-rating scale? Before evaluating the evidence, it should be noted that the test-retest reliabilities of loudness matching and self-report loudness scales have not yet been properly established (McFadden 1982, Hallam et al 1986). A correlation between the two variables cannot exceed the reliability coefficient of either measure (unless error variance is correlated), and it is likely to be a good deal lower. Therefore, evidence of absent or low correlations cannot readily be accepted at the present time. Moreover, authors of relevant papers have not given sufficient information about the way the self-rating scales have been constructed or administered, or whether, for example, the loudness judgement refers to the loudness of the tinnitus in general or the loudness at a particular time under particular listening conditions. Ideally, of course, the conditions should duplicate those in which the loudness match is made. The evidence shows that the correlation coefficient rarely exceeds 0.4 to 0.5 (whether the loudness match is expressed in HL, SPL, SL, PLU or sones) and that different authors get different results with similar methods (Reed 1960, Hazell 1981b, Tyler & Conrad-Armes 1983, Hallam et al 1986). Loudness as measured by matching and self-report may, in fact, reflect different aspects of tinnitus 'intensity' and discrepancies between the two measures may be of clinical interest, as others have noted (Hazell 1981, Taylor & Conrad Armes 1983). However, recent work by the author and his colleagues suggests that the correlation may be appreciably affected by measurement problems, such as the failure of subjects to perform the judgement tasks adequately (Jakes et al 1986). With an improved self-rating methodology and the exclusion of subjects who had difficulty in carrying our either the loudness match or the self-rating, the correlation coefficient between loudness-match values expressed in PLUs and a Guttman scale of reported loudness rose to 0.73. Improvement in quantitative techniques should permit future research to proceed on a sounder basis.

Studies of the relationship between loudness match and measures of distress/handicap obviously suffer from similar problems. The association is generally low. Mean loudness match values were found to be no different for complaining and non-complaining tinnitus patients (Hallam et al 1984). The correlation coefficient between several self-report measures of distress and loudness match expressed in PLUs have been found to be statistically significant but generally low and of the order of 0.40 to 0.50 (Hallam et al 1986). It might be the case that the correlation differs between complaining and non-complaining subjects. In other words, when any complaint about tinnitus is registered, its 'intensity' may become a salient and determining factor. For essentially non-complaining subjects tinnitus intensity may be less important.

At this point it should be noted that tinnitus complaint has not yet been adequately defined. If, as I suggested earlier, complaint is likely to be multi-dimensional, it is possible that different dimensions of complaint relate in different ways to the several sensory features of tinnitus noises. Work on tinnitus complaint will now be reviewed.

THE NATURE OF TINNITUS DISTRESS AND ANNOYANCE

As previously mentioned, epidemiological studies indicate that only a fraction of those individuals who report tinnitus actually complain that it disturbs their daily life. This is just as well because tinnitus is such a common phenomenon. Even so, it is estimated that in 5% of the British adult population sleep is disturbed by tinnitus (Coles et al 1981). Of course, this figure is based on people's judgements that this is true for them. It is not a statement of causality. It is up to the clinician to assess the causes of symptoms and apportion distress to different causative factors. This assessment can be very difficult to make in some tinnitus sufferers. For example, a high proportion of patients in whom tinnitus is a chronic and severe complaint are judged to be clinically depressed. Estimates range from 20 to 50% (see House 1981). Hazell, in the discussion of House's paper, noted that about half of depressed tinnitus sufferers have a long history of depressive illness before tinnitus starts. House reported an 80% improvement rate with biofeedback training and noted that depressed patients improved most of all. This suggests that depressive mood is often secondary to the stress of tinnitus noises. However, it is also likely that the supportive counselling she provided in addition to biofeedback effectively tackled long-standing psychological problems which preceded tinnitus onset. For example, she states that, at the outset, patients had to be persuaded to see their tinnitus in psychological terms, but that at the finish, 80% reported more understanding of the effects of the emotions on bodily functions and 40% sought further counselling or psychotherapy.

These observations highlight the difficulty that may be encountered in establishing the causes and consequences of tinnitus. The undesirability of classifying patients as either primarily 'medical' or 'psychiatric' has already been mentioned. The aim of the present section is to analyse the complaints of the tinnitus sufferer in greater detail, thereby easing the tasks of assessing and apportioning distress. It is likely that different therapeutic approaches will be required for different tinnitus complaints, tailored to suit the individual's needs. It is a temptation for patient and clinician alike to attribute distress to the most obvious symptom, namely tinnitus. On even superficial examination, this may be shown to be false or, at most, tinnitus is found to be an additional or interactive factor. For example, tinnitus sufferers complaining of sleep disturbance might always have been poor sleepers. As noted above, depressed or anxious mood often precedes the onset of tinnitus. This is not to deny that in altered mood states, attention to tinnitus noises can form the focus of worries or of a sense of helplessness. However, in these circumstances, the clinician is wrong in restricting attention to the tinnitus symptom itself.

Furthermore, tinnitus is commonly associated with other otological symptoms such as hearing loss, dizziness and unsteadiness. Patients may be unaware of hearing loss and blame all their hearing difficulties on tinnitus. Others complain of difficulty in hearing which may be attributable to intrusive tinnitus noise. These confusions are fairly readily detected during the audiometric assessment but the implication of their resolution may be far-reaching for the patient.

Recent studies have demonstrated the importance of complaints of dizziness in the distress experienced by tinnitus sufferers (Hallam & Stephens 1986, Stephens & Hallam 1986). Emotional distress was measured by means of a psychopathology questionnaire which can be scored on different dimensions (The Crown–Crisp Experiential Index, CCEI) (Crown & Crisp 1979). A group of patients whose main complaint was tinnitus was divided into those who also complained of dizziness, hearing difficulty, or both. Tinnitus as a sole complaint was associated with elevated scores on the 'free-floating-anxiety' and 'depression' scales compared to population norms. When tinnitus patients complained also of dizziness this was associated with higher scores on 'somatic anxiety' and 'phobic anxiety'. The presence of hearing difficulty (and/or an elevated hearing threshold) bore no relationship to CCEI scores. These findings imply that emotional distress in tinnitus patients may be related to other symptoms, especially dizziness. However, a puzzling feature of the results of the study of Hallam & Stephens (1986) was that the complaint of dizziness was unrelated to the results of behavioural tests of balance. It might be the case that the symptom of dizziness is simply one of a number of other anxiety complaints. This is unlikely to be the whole explanation because subjects were attending a neuro-otology clinic and the physician judged, without seeing the results of the balance tests, that a proportion were in fact suffering some degree of vertigo or unsteadiness. It is uncertain as to whether the psychological characteristics associated with the combined complaint of dizziness and tinnitus are unrelated to neuro-otological disorders, or whether these disorders bring them about through a somatopsychic effect (see e.g. Hinchcliffe 1983).

Tension headache is another complaint which is commonly associated with tinnitus. A number of clinicians have noted that tinnitus can lead to muscular tension in the head and neck region which in turn produces headache. In some individuals, tinnitus is perceived as 'boring through the head' or 'filling the head with pressure'. The phenomenology of tinnitus therefore merges with that of headache.

In summary, the sources of emotional distress in tinnitus patients are likely to be multifactorial and include factors unrelated to tinnitus *per se*. However, some tinnitus suffering is quite specifically associated with features of the tinnitus such as its intrusiveness in certain situations. Evidence concerning the more specific effects is reviewed below.

Specific difficulties and worries experienced by tinnitus sufferers

Until recently, evidence on the way tinnitus affects a person's life was largely anecdotal. In order to document the problems of tinnitus sufferers, Tyler & Baker (1983) asked members of a self-help association for tinnitus to list in order of importance, their main difficulties resulting from tinnitus. The average number of difficulties for the respondents who replied (74%) was between four and five. Respondents who had had tinnitus for the shortest period of time reported the largest range of problems. Life-style was affected in 90%, the most frequent effect being 'difficulty getting to sleep' (57%). Emotional problems were mentioned by 70% and these included despair, frustration, depression, irritation, inability to relax, difficulty in concentration, confusion and worry. Difficulties in relation to health and health care were mentioned by 56%, the most frequent being dependence on drugs (24%) followed by pain/headaches (18%). Effects on hearing were noted by 53% of the sample, the most common of which was understanding speech (37%).

The difficulties with the highest importance rating (tending to be ranked first) were 'getting to sleep', 'family problems' and 'persistence of tinnitus'. The latter is not so much a difficulty but presumably refers to an inability to turn attention away from the noises. The sample was an elderly one (mean age 62 years) which might explain the slight mention of interference with work (4%). Some of the hearing difficulties that were reported could, of couse, have interfered with work efficiency. Some respondents avoided quiet situations if their tinnitus was noticeably worse in these instances, whereas others avoided noisy situations.

It may not be possible to generalize these findings to all tinnitus sufferers, given that this sample consisted of people sufficiently troubled to join a self-help association, and some difficulties may be attributable to hearing loss. Nevertheless, the difficulties are consistent with anecdotal descriptions in the clinical literature and indicate that for many people tinnitus is by no means a trivial problem.

It is natural to ask how the difficulties experienced by individuals who complain of tinnitus differ from those who do not complain and whether this difference is related to the personality characteristics of the sufferer, the severity of the difficulties or the type of difficulty. A pilot investigation of this type was performed with clinic patients (Hallam et al 1984). The non-complaining patients were attending on account of other otological symptoms but also reported tinnitus on questioning. Neither tinnitus loudness match or rated loudness was related to complaint but differences on some self-report scales underlined the importance of some of the difficulties discovered by Tyler & Baker (1983). Complainers described the noises as more persistent and they were more aware of them. There was greater interference with work, with hearing in group situations, and with sleep onset. The complainers also described themselves as more depressed, they had consulted doctors to a greater degree and used more psychotropic drugs.

In a further series of studies by the author and his colleagues, techniques of factor analysis were employed to examine the association between different tinnitus problems and worries. The analyses were designed to show whether tinnitus complaints could be conceived as unidimensional or whether complaints grouped themselves into several independent dimensions. In two studies (one unpublished) of complaining tinnitus patients attending a specialist out-patient clinic, complaint behaviour was found to be multidimensional. The items used in the first analyses (Jakes et al 1986) included self-ratings on category scales of various qualitative features of tinnitus noises and their effect on daily life as well as hearing difficulties and symptoms of vestibular disorders. Audiometric measures (pitch and loudness matching, hearing thresholds, minimal masking level, etc) were also included in the analyses. To summarise the results, tinnitus complaint factors were found to be independent of hearing difficulty and vestibular symptoms, and with minor exceptions, self-reported tinnitus complaints did not cluster with any of the audiometric measures. The principal tinnitus complaint factors are tabulated in Table 9.1. (Other factors derived from the analysis are not tabulated – see Jakes et al 1986). They were labelled 'emotional distress', 'intrusiveness', 'interference with passive auditory entertainment', 'intensity of tinnitus' and 'sleep disturbance'. Some of these factors are loaded by only a few items and their existence must be regarded as questionable until replicated.

It is of considerable interest that the intrusiveness of tinnitus (how loud, distracting and unpleasant it is) forms a factor which is independent of emotional distress.

Table 9.1 Tinnitus complaint factors in first factor analysis (orthogonal varimax solution, $n=82$). Figures refer to item loadings

Emotional distress (13% of variance)	
Family and social life affected	0.85
Irritability	0.68
Depressed	0.62
Work affected	0.60
Not coping	0.50
Use of tranquillizers	0.32
Intrusiveness (11% of variance)	
Self-reported loudness	0.76
Distracted by tinnitus	0.76
Tinnitus unpleasant	0.70
Not coping	0.42
Interference with passive auditory entertainment (7% of variance)	
Listening to music	0.84
Watching TV	0.81
Intensity of tinnitus (6% of variance)	
Loudness match SL (tinnitus frequency)	0.77
Loudness match SL (1kHz)	0.66
Minimal masking level (HL)	0.39
Uncomfortable loudness level	0.38
Age	0.38
Sleep disturbance (6% of variance)	
Middle insomnia	0.74
Early insomnia	0.70
Sex	0.37

However, both factors are loaded by an item measuring difficulty in coping. The sleep disturbance factor also forms a separate factor (see Jakes et al 1986 for a discussion of these findings).

Our second study (unpublished) employed a new questionnaire composed of 40 statements about the effects of tinnitus culled from interviews with patients. No audiometric measures were included. Three main tinnitus complaint factors were obtained (see Table 9.2). The largest concerned emotional distress as in the first analysis. The content of the items strongly suggest that distress was related to worries about physical and mental health. The second factor was composed of items reflecting auditory perceptual problems, especially listening to speech. These difficulties may be unrelated to hearing thresholds in any direct way and the factor may correspond to the 'intrusiveness' factor of the first analysis, which, it should be noted, was independent of a hearing difficulty factor. Once more, items indicative of sleep disturbance clustered together and formed a separate factor.

Table 9.2 Tinnitus complaint factors in second factor analysis (orthogonal varimax solution, $n=79$). Figures refer to item loadings.

Emotional distress (40% of variance)	
I worry that there is something seriously wrong with my body	0.76
I worry that the noises might damage my physical health	0.72
Life seems to be getting on top of me	0.67
I am more concerned about my health	0.66
I worry that the noises will give me a nervous breakdown	0.61
I worry whether I will be able to put up with this problem forever	0.58
I have lost some of my confidence	0.57
I find it harder to relax	0.52
I am liable to feel low	0.48
Auditory perceptual problems (15% of variance)	
I have more difficulty in telling where sounds are coming from	0.74
I find it harder to use the phone	0.71
Voices sound distorted to me	0.71
It is more difficult to listen to several people at once	0.64
I have more difficulty following a conversation	0.57
Sleep disturbance (7% of variance)	
I wake up more in the night	0.73
I wake up earlier in the morning	0.67
It takes me longer to get to sleep	0.60

The implications of the multidimensional nature of tinnitus complaint behaviour are: 1. That a global concept of tinnitus 'severity' may not be all that meaningful and ideally, severity measures should refer to single dimensions of complaint; 2. That in any evaluation of tinnitus treatments there should be an attempt to quantify the separate facets of disturbance by tinnitus. A more specific implication is that treatments may effectively modify one aspect of disturbance (e.g. sleep) but not another. It has been widely reported that measures of tinnitus 'intensity' (e.g. loudness match) are unrelated to other tinnitus complaints or improvement after therapy but with a more sophisticated breakdown of complaint, this generalisation may not hold up. Our first analysis indicated that intensity measures are unrelated to the major factor of emotional distress. However, self-ratings of loudness would appear to relate to intrusiveness (see Table 9.1) which, in turn, may be associated with certain auditory perceptual difficulties rather than distress.

It remains to be seen whether the tinnitus complaint dimensions are associated with any of the broader categories of 'psychopathology' which are frequently mentioned in descriptive accounts of tinnitus patients. For example, do patients who worry about tinnitus also worry about other somatic symptoms or is a feeling of helplessness associated with tinnitus also indicative of a general inability to cope with daily problems? We have obtained some evidence that specific worries and distress attributed to tinnitus are positively correlated with scores on a psychopathology questionnaire (Stephens & Hallam 1986) but the correlations were low. It is our impression that the majority of tinnitus sufferers do not have generalised psychological difficulties of which tinnitus is just one symptomatic expression.

PSYCHOLOGICAL APPROACHES TO MANAGEMENT

A variety of therapies have been attempted with tinnitus sufferers. The rationale underlying each therapy often varies more than the techniques themselves. As we have seen, complaints about tinnitus are not unidimensional and some variation in approach according to presenting problems must surely be recommended. If tinnitus is thought to be associated with severe anxiety or depression or seen as serving a function in the individual's interpersonal relationships, then therapy aimed solely at alleviating tinnitus distress would not be expected to prove very beneficial.

The fact that diverse methods such as electrical stimulation (Chouard et al 1981), dietary changes (Yanick 1981) and relaxation exercises (Grossan 1976) benefit at least some patients should alert researchers to the potency of non-specific components of therapy and the need for controlled evaluation trials.

Psychological interventions should form part of an integrated approach to tinnitus management (see Stephens 1984; Dr. Stephens is evolving a preliminary systems model). Drug therapies and the use of maskers are not reviewed here (see McFadden 1982), and Chs. 10 and 5 in this volume).

It might be predicted from the habituation model presented earlier that different therapies exert benefit through a common pathway. For example, therapy might persuade the individual to adopt a different mental set towards the noises, to worry less about them, or to cope differently when bothered by them. These changes might be expected to facilitate the habituation of attention to the noises. Of course, this process is expected to occur spontaneously and so the sheer passage of time should be accompanied by a certain amount of relief.

The outcome of therapy cannot be evaluated without regard for the characteristics of the sample of patients. Recent onset cases should show considerable improvement with the passage of time and with non-specific attention and reassurance. However, when tinnitus has been present for 18 months or more and other treatments have failed, even low rates of improvement can be clinically significant. Unfortunately, not all studies give sufficient details of their subjects' characteristics. The term 'severe tinnitus', as noted earlier, lacks precision and suffers from implying unidimensionality of tinnitus complaint.

This section aims to evaluate the contribution of psychological therapies to tinnitus management. The aim of these therapies is to reduce distress and disablement but not to 'cure' tinnitus. However, if a patient is no longer troubled by tinnitus and there are no discernible effects on the quality of life, it may be of little consequence whether tinnitus is present or not. Many millions of people appear to tolerate it without undue concern. There is no doubt that tinnitus has a physiological or pathophysiological basis. It is not a psychiatric or psychological disorder and so the question as to whether or not there is an effective psychological treatment should not arise. Having said this, some crude improvement figures can be provided for a number of 'shotgun' approaches. To begin with, it is interesting to examine improvement rates with non-specific (placebo) therapies in order to provide a reference level for evaluation.

Erlandsson and her colleagues (1983, 1986) compared a masking instrument and an identical-looking placebo device which the patient was told delivered a weak (subliminal) electrical shock. Subjects who were 'severely disturbed' by tinnitus received six weeks of each treatment in a cross-over design. Intensity of tinnitus was rated daily. Five out of 17 subjects (29%) gained significant improvement from both devices. Overall, the groups did not differ in terms of mean change on the diary measure. Three were improved by maskers only and none by placebo only. Thus, a placebo effect appeared to be operating, with only a slight superiority being shown by the masking treatment (maskers were, incidentally, said to confer some additional advantages over placebo treatment).

In a study comparing acupuncture and placebo acupuncture in a double-blind cross-over trial, patients with tinnitus of at least one year's duration and otherwise resistant to treatment were found to benefit equally from both (Hansen et al 1982). Only one of the tinnitus groups (placebo followed by acupuncture) showed a significant decline in tinnitus 'intensity' over the treatment period but the absence of any other measures of outcome makes it difficult to draw any conclusions about the effectiveness of treatment. In a very similar study (Marks et al 1984) the brief nature of the acupuncture and the limited range of measures of outcome make it difficult to draw any conclusions about the benefits of acupuncture of placebo acupuncture. However, following acupuncture five of the 14 patients reported some positive changes, whereas none did following placebo treatment.

Relaxation and stress-management

These approaches have been employed to modify the patient's emotional response to the tinnitus noises. Some authors see muscle relaxation as a way of reducing anxiety in general: the less generally anxious a person is, the less likely, it is assumed, will he respond emotionally to tinnitus. Grossan (1976) also believes that tinnitus distress causes spastic contraction of neck muscles with consequent headache and altered circulation in the ear. Muscle relaxation is therefore viewed as having a specific effect in alleviating tinnitus suffering. House (1978) combined biofeedback training (to reduce frontalis muscle EMG and increase body temperature) with relaxation exercises. The aim was to help the patient discriminate physiological functions associated with 'stress' and to reduce them by achieving a relaxed state. House also stated that tinnitus is perceived as being louder when the subject is tense. On this view, relaxation training also brings about a perceptual change. Some support for this idea was obtained by Malatesta et al (1980) in a single case study.

Grossan (1976) offered EMG (frontalis muscle) biofeedback training to 66 patients of whom 51 accepted. Various instructions to induce relaxation were also given. The patients were said to have been unresponsive to previous treatments but over 80% reported subjective improvement with biofeedback, though it is difficult, on the information provided, to know what this meant in practice. Loudness match measures showed no systematic change.

House (1978) reported the results of biofeedback plus relaxation training in

41 patients who had failed with other methods of treatment. Fifteen (36%) were much, or very much, improved after 12 sessions. At 6–12 month follow-up only 7 remained in this category although 16 had slight improvement. Assessment was by global questionnaire ratings. Despite the modest gains, 25 patients noted an increased awareness of the effects of tension on bodily state and its relationship to their perception of tinnitus sensations. This awareness was apparently associated with a change of attitude towards tinnitus and this had generally beneficial effects. It seems that a large number of patients rejected biofeedback or dropped out of therapy because they saw their tinnitus in strictly medical terms (House 1978). Of those who persisted, about 40% sought further counselling or psychotherapy. Biofeedback, as a quasi-medical technology, may be a useful way of helping patients to see that psychological factors are relevant, if this is a new idea to them. There is, perhaps, little point in attempting any psychological approach in patients who do not see their problem in these terms at all.

In some applications of relaxation training, it is considered that relaxation can be compared to an acquired skill which the patient can apply when the noises are particularly distressing. Tinnitus noise itself has been suggested as a cue to apply the relaxation skill (e.g. Grossan 1976).

Marlowe (1973) used hypnotic techniques with two tinnitus sufferers, suggesting to one of them that relaxation and diminished tinnitus intensity would later be associated with attention to tinnitus noises. In the second case, relaxation was induced hypnotically together with the suggestion that mental state could modify physical symptoms. A post-hypnotic suggestion was given to the effect that a pleasant piece of music would appear whenever he became aware of his tinnitus. Tinnitus annoyance and sleep disturbance decreased in both cases.

A similar combination of hypnotic suggestion, relaxation training and imagery was tried by Macleod Morgan et al (1982) who referred to their technique as 'cognitive restructuring'. One patient was instructed to seek out her 'hum' to use it as a cue for relaxation. The technique was facilitated by the mental image of turning down a control knob. Similar imagery was used to good effect in two other cases. In collaboration with the subject, images were chose to be particularly pleasant and to permit some imaginary control of the noise. In this way, it was intended that the noises be 'accepted' without self-defeating efforts to control their presence.

Lyndberg and colleagues (1984) adopted the method of 'applied relaxation' combined with 'perceptual restructuring' in treating a single case. The patient was first taught how to relax on cue and finally to apply relaxation when imagining situations that provoked distress attributed to tinnitus. When relaxed, he switched to pleasant imagery. These techniques were practised in the actual situations (at work) when tinnitus was troublesome. Ratings of tinnitus annoyance and also level (i.e. intensity) were made four times daily. Annoyance dropped 71% between baseline and follow-up and tinnitus level dropped 20%. Some general benefits of therapy were also observed.

In a systematic evaluation of these techniques, 24 patients complaining of tinnitus for at least one year and who were generally unresponsive to other treatments received applied relaxation training and perceptual restructuring (Scott et al 1986). Ten sessions were given over two to three weeks. The loudness of the tinnitus was rated four times daily and retrospectively at the end of the day. Depression and irritability were also rated on a daily basis. As described above, the technique consisted of teaching the subject to relax to a cue word, and instructing him or her to apply it in situations where tinnitus distress was provoked. When relaxed the subject switched attention to a pleasant scene. When relaxed the subject switched attention to a pleasant scene. As training progressed, the technique was practised in increasingly provocative tinnitus-distress situations (special efforts were made to identify these in the initial interviews). The extent to which the therapist prompted attention-switching and self-control decreased as training went on.

A delayed treatment group was used as an experimental control. These subjects made daily recordings while awaiting treatment. The results indicated a significant reduction in tinnitus level, discomfort arising from the tinnitus, and in depression in the experimental group only. The two groups shared a significant reduction on almost all outcome measures except the psychoacoustic ones; the greatest change was observed on depression and discomfort. Thirteen out of 21 subjects were judged to show definite all-round improvement and four showed none at all. There were no systematic changes in psychoacoustic measures.

Value of psychological therapies

A variety of techniques reduce distress in at least some tinnitus patients and this emphasises the need for controlled trials. There is little or no evidence for loudness match values declining after any of the treatments reviewed above. With the exception of a few studies, the outcome measures employed have been inadequate to test the hypothesis that distress or annoyance (rather than, say, self-rated loudness) declines with therapy. In one subject in whom mood disturbance and phobias were successfully treated by psychological means (Hallam & Jakes 1986) there was a clear reduction in tinnitus distress but little change in measures of tinnitus intrusiveness, loudness ratings, or loudness match values. Scott and her colleagues (1986) also reported greater change in 'discomfort' ratings than in 'level' (intensity) ratings, and no systematic change on psychoacoustic variables at all.

The lack of impact of psychological techniques on intensity measures of tinnitus should not distract from their positive effects on distress and annoyance. It is the latter, after all, which tend to lead the patient to seek help. The mechanism by which these positive effects are brought about is far from clear and may well be different for different individuals. The therapies that have so far been investigated contain a variety of components, and the subjects in these trials do not form a homogenous group. Mechanisms can only be elucidated by categorising subjects according to the precise nature of their complaints and by systematically varying treatment components. Present results indicate that this kind of research effort would be worthwhile. As a general recommendation, it may be stated that counselling and relaxation (whether applied by means of biofeedback or hypnosis or taught as a stress-management strategy) are useful approaches in cases of chronic and unrelenting tinnitus annoyance. An approach involving group meetings which nevertheless stresses the specific nature of individuals' maladaptive attitudes and coping strategies appears to be very promising (Sweetow 1984). The groups make use of cognitive-behavioural modification principles, originally developed for chronic pain patients. A proportion of tinnitus sufferers have psychological problems in addition to those arising out of tinnitus and the services of appropriate mental health professionals should then be sought.

Psychological approaches to evaluation and management

The importance of emotional and other psychological factors in managing the tinnitus patient was sensitively discussed by Fowler and Fowler (1955)–a paper which still deserves to be read. A psychological approach to the tinnitus patient has been recognised as one component of an integrated model of management (see Coles 1983, Stephens 1984). The overall evaluation of the patient will of course include assessing both tinnitus and hearing and their interrelationship, the role of environmental noise in producing either relief or exacerbation of distress, patient's general expectations and beliefs regarding tinnitus, and so on. The typical neuro-otology clinic or auditory rehabilitation centre may not have the services of a mental health professional skilled in evaluating the psychological contribution to the patient's complaints. However, complaint questionnaires (Jakes et al 1986) and standardised tests of psychological status may be of value. The initial evaluation, which should include the following questions, is not in any case a mental health evaluation. Broadly speaking, the most relevant questions are:

1. Is tinnitus a source of annoyance or distress? (If not, explanation, reassurance, and treatment of underlying causes where possible, should suffice)
2. Are there signs that the patient is developing tolerance of the noises? (If so, then the patient may be reassured that this process should continue, and be reviewed later)
3. Is only a medical cure acceptable to the patient? (If so, the role of psychological factors can be explained, the patient reassured and reviewed later)
4. Is further attention to tinnitus likely to be counter-productive? (If so, medical or psychological treatment might simply reinforce the seriousness of the disorder in the patient's eyes and confirm existing health concerns)

In a number of patients, distress and annoyance persist despite the explanation and reassurance provided by the clinician. Where the distress is clearly related to tinnitus onset and to situations in which tinnitus is more distressing because of tinnitus-related factors, then some of the psychological approaches reviewed above (or pharmacological approaches) may be considered. When insomnia is the most prominent complaint, relaxation methods are especially appropriate.

Some patients will be judged as having psychological problems which even though associated with tinnitus (as discussed earlier) essentially require treatment in their own right. Referral to an appropriate mental health professional to assess and/or treat these problems is then recommended. Successful resolution of the problem can lead to a significant reduction of tinnitus distress (Hallam & Jakes 1986).

There are a small number of tinnitus sufferers for whom all current approaches are unsuccessful. For these unfortunate people, supportive and pharmacological therapies are likely to remain the mainstay of management.

Acknowledgements

This chapter has been greatly improved by incorporating the comments and suggestions of R Hinchcliffe, S Jakes and S D G Stephens. The author is supported by the Medical Research Council of Great Britain.

REFERENCES

Chouard C H, Meyer B, Maridat D 1981 Transcutaneous electrotherapy for severe tinnitus. Acta Otolaryngologica 91: 415–422
Coles R R A 1984 Measurement and management of tinnitus. Proceedings of the Tinnitus Seminar, Uppsala, Nov 1983. Swedish Council for Planning and Coordination of Research
Coles R R A, Davis A C, Haggard M P 1981 Epidemiology of tinnitus. In: Evered D, Lawrenson G (eds) Tinnitus. Ciba Foundation Symposium 85. Pitman, London, pp 16–34
Crown S, Crisp A H 1979 Manual of the Crown-Crisp Experiential Index. Hodder and Stoughton, London
Erlandsson S 1984 Behandling med masker och placebo-effekter. Proceedings of the Tinnitus Seminar, Uppsala, Nov 1983. Swedish Council for Planning and Coordination of Research
Erlandsson S, Ringdahl A, Hutchins T, Carlsson S G 1986 Treatment of tinnitus: a controlled comparison of masking and placebo. Scandinavian Audiology (in press)
Fowler E P 1936 Head noises; significance, measurement, and importance in diagnosis and treatment. Archives of Otolaryngology 24: 731–741
Fowler E P, Fowler E P 1955 Somatopsychic and psychosomatic factors in tinnitus, deafness and vertigo. Annals of Otology, Rhinology and Laryngology 64: 29–37
Goodwin P E, Johnson R M 1980 The loudness of tinnitus. Acta Otolaryngologica 90: 353–359
Grossan M 1976 Treatment of subjective tinnitus with biofeedback. Ear Nose and Throat Journal 55: 314–318
Hallam R S, Jakes S C 1985 Tinnitus: Differential effects of therapy in a single case. Behaviour Research and Therapy, 6: 691–694
Hallam R S, Stephens S D G 1985 Vestibular disorder and emotional distress. Journal of Psychosomatic Research 29: 407–413
Hallam R S, Rachman S, Hinchcliffe R 1984 Psychological aspects of tinnitus. In: Rachman S (ed) Contributions to medical psychology, Vol 3, Pergamon, Oxford, pp 31–34
Hallam R S, Jakes S C, Chambers C, Hinchcliffe R 1986 A comparison of different methods for assessing the 'intensity' of tinnitus. Acta Otolaryngologica 99: 501–508
Hansen P E, Hansen J H, Bentzen O 1982 Acupuncture treatment of chronic unilateral tinnitus: a double blind crossover trial. Clinical Otolaryngology 7: 325–329
Hazell J W P 1981a Patterns of tinnitus: medical audiological findings. In: Proceedings of the First International Tinnitus Seminar, New York, 1979. Journal of Laryngology and Otology, Supplement 4
Hazell J W P 1981b Measurement of tinnitus in humans. In: Evered D, Lawrenson G (eds) Tinnitus. Ciba Foundation Symposium 85, Pitman, London, pp 35–53
Heller M F, Bergmann M 1953 Tinnitus aurium in normally hearing persons. Annals of Otology Rhinology and Laryngology 62: 73–83
Hinchcliffe R 1961 Prevalence of the commoner ear, nose and throat conditions in the adult rural population of Great Britain. British Journal of Preventative and Social Medicine 15: 128–140
Hinchcliffe R 1983 Psychological and sociological facets of balance disorders. In: Hinchcliffe R (ed) Hearing and balance in the elderly. Churchill Livingstone, Edinburgh, pp 453–467
Hinchcliffe R, Chambers C 1983 Loudness of tinnitus: an approach to measurement. Advances in Oto-Rhino-Laryngology 29: 163–173
House J W 1978 Treatment of severe tinnitus with biofeedback training. Laryngoscope 88: 406–412

House P R 1981 Personality of the tinnitus patient. In: Evered D, Lawrenson G (eds) Tinnitus. Ciba Foundation Symposium 85, Pitman, London, pp 193–203
Jakes S C, Hallam R S, Chambers C, Hinchcliffe R 1985 A factor analytical study of tinnitus complaint behaviour. Audiology 24: 195–206
Lyndberg P, Lyttkens L, Melin L, Scott B 1984 The use of a coping technique in the treatment of tinnitus. Scandinavian Journal of Behaviour Therapy 13: 117–121
McFadden D 1982 Tinnitus: facts, theories and treatments. Working Group 89, National Research Council, Washington DC, National Academy Press, Washington
McLeod Morgan C, Court J, Roberts R 1982 Cognitive restructuring: a technique for the relief of chronic tinnitus. Australian Journal of Clinical and Experimental Hypnosis 10: 27–33
Malatesta V J, Sutker P B, Adams H E 1980 Experimental assessment of tinnitus aurium. Journal of Behavioural Assessment 2: 309–317
Marks N J, Emery P, Onisiphorou C 1984 A controlled trial of acupuncture in tinnitus. Journal of Laryngology and Otology 98: 1103–1109
Marlowe F I 1973 Effective treatment of tinnitus through hypnotherapy. American Journal of Clinical Hypnosis 15: 162–165
Mitchell C 1983 The masking of tinnitus with pure tones. Audiology 22: 73–87
Office of Population Censuses and Surveys 1983 General Household Survey: the prevalence of tinnitus 1981. OPCS Monitor GHS 83/1. OPCS, London
Penner M J, Brauth S, Hood L 1981 The temporal course of the masking of tinnitus as a basis for inferring its origin. Journal of Speech and Hearing Research 24: 257–261
Reed G F 1960 An audiometric study of 200 cases of subjective tinnitus. Archives of Otolaryngology 71: 94–104
Reich G E, Johnson R M 1984 Personality characteristics of tinnitus patients. Journal of Laryngology and Otology, Supplement 9: 228–232
Scott B, Lindberg P, Lyttkens L, Melin L 1985 Psychological treatment of tinnitus. Scandinavian Audiology 14: 223–230
Stephens S D G 1986 The management of tinnitus. Paper to the International Workshop Symposium on Neuro-otology, Asiago, Italy, January 1984. Audiologia Italiana (in press)
Stephens S D G, Corcoran A 1985 A controlled study of tinnitus masking. British Journal of Audiology 19: 159–167
Stephens S D G, Hallam R S 1985 The Crown-Crisp Experiential Index in patients complaining of tinnitus. British Journal of Audiology 19: 151–158
Sweetow R W 1984 Cognitive-behavioural modification in tinnitus management. Hearing Instruments 35(9): 14–18, 52
Tyler R S, Baker L J 1983 Difficulties experienced by tinnitus sufferers. Journal of Speech and Hearing Disorders 48: 150–154
Tyler R S, Conrad-Armes D 1983 The determination of tinnitus loudness considering the effects of recruitment. Journal of Speech and Hearing Research 26: 59–72
Walford R E 1979 People who hear a continuous hum. Science Chelsea, 8(3): 7–9
Yanick P 1981 Tinnitus–an holistic approach. Hearing Instruments 32(7): 12–15, 39

10

R. J. Goodey

Drug therapy in tinnitus

For any condition a simple and reliable drug remedy has great appeal both to the patient and to the busy clinician. There is no longer any doubt that tinnitus can sometimes be suppressed by drugs. However, the use of these drugs is not simple nor are the responses to them consistent. Indeed the same drug which can ameliorate tinnitus in one patient may cause or aggravate it in another, tinnitus being a symptom which may result from a variety of disorders and mechanisms. Nevertheless for some patients tinnitus is so distressing that a clinician dealing with these severe cases should be familiar with and able to utilise drug therapy when appropriate.

Drug therapies to suppress tinnitus must be distinguished from specific therapies for specific disorders for which tinnitus is one of the symptoms. Thus tinnitus may be eased when infections are treated with antibiotics or immunological disorders with steroids; when Ménière's disease or Paget's disease is stabilised; when vitamin, mineral or hormone deficiencies are replaced and depressive and anxiety states controlled. There is a temptation for a clinician who has been delighted with the tinnitus relief resulting from specific treatment of a particular disorder to use the same treatment for other patients with tinnitus irrespective of the associated disorder.

LITERATURE REVIEW

Local anaesthetic agents

Barany (1936) reported temporary relief from tinnitus after injection of local anaesthetic into nasal turbinates. Lewy (1937) and Englesson et al (1976) deliberately used intravenous local anaesthetic to treat tinnitus and Gejrot (1963, 1976) and Fowler (1953) noted relief from tinnitus while treating acute episodes of Ménière's disease with intravenous local anaesthetics. In 1975 anaesthetists at the Auckland Pain Clinic noted that patients injected with lignocaine (lidocaine) intravenously, to test whether their pain was of central origin (Hatangdi et al 1976) sometimes received temporary relief from coincidental tinnitus. This observation led Melding et al (1978) to study the effects of intravenous lignocaine on patients with tinnitus which was considered both incurable and intolerable. Responses were correlated with independent audiometric and clinical assessment. Of 78 patients 63% experienced between 60% and total relief from tinnitus. Of 41 patients in whom hearing loss and tinnitus were independently attributed to damage to the organ of Corti, the proportion gaining comparable relief rose to 85%.

Shea and Harell (1978) and Shea et al (1981) were quick to confirm and extend the New Zealand experience. Emmett (1981) reported from the Shea Clinic that of 590 patients with bilateral tinnitus and 783 patients with unilateral tinnitus, 60% to 80% achieved between 50% and 100% relief with intravenous lignocaine. Martin & Colman (1980) in a double-blind cross-over controlled trial confirmed the effectiveness of intravenous lignocaine while noting the short duration of action. Israel et al (1982) in a placebo-controlled double-blind cross-over study found 19 out of 26 patients reported subjective tinnitus better or gone with intravenous lignocaine and that there was no change with saline. Majumdar et al (1983) with 20 patients found 13 improved with intravenous lignocaine and only three with saline controls. Jackson (1981) confirmed that where the tinnitus responded to intravenous lignocaine the amount of relief varied as did the serum level. In trials with similar but longer-acting agents he found that bupivacaine did not give a longer action as anticipated; intravenous lorcainide did produce relief for as long as eight hours but was followed by intolerable sleep disturbance. Causse et al (1984) report momentary reduction of severe and decompensated tinnitus following injection of the local anaesthetic Renovaine into the external ear canal.

Duckert & Rees (1983) conducted a double-blind randomised trial to assess the effectiveness of intravenous lignocaine on tinnitus. Of the lignocaine group 40% had decreased tinnitus and 30% increased tinnitus. The present author had also noted (Goodey 1981) that while intravenous lignocaine could temporarily reduce or abolish tinnitus in many patients it could aggravate existing tinnitus in some. This led him to propose intravenous lignocaine as a test to distinguish patients whose tinnitus may be helped by drugs with an action similar to lignocaine from those whose tinnitus may be caused or aggravated by such drugs, which should therefore be looked for and withdrawn.

Melding et al (1978) had concluded that intravenous lignocaine is highly effective in suppressing tinnitus in patients with damage or degeneration of the organ of Corti but not in other groups. After reviewing analogous situations they suggested that in these patients tinnitus is due to abnormal hyperactivity in the central auditory pathways, the hyperactivity being due either to increased excitability or to release from inhibitory mechanisms. Intravenous lignocaine, a known membrane stabiliser, was presumed to relieve the tinnitus by blocking the abnormal hyperactivity. This concept led Melding & Goodey (1979) to a trial of oral anticonvulsants for relief of tinnitus in patients who had gained temporary relief with lignocaine. The observation that in some patients tinnitus is aggravated by intravenous lignocaine (Goodey 1981, Duckert & Rees 1983) suggests that in these patients the mechanism may be a reduction in the spontaneous activity in the auditory pathways. Other possible mechanisms which might be influenced by drugs would include abnormal activity arising in the cochlea itself and crosstalk due to abnormal phase locking of spontaneous activity between damaged neurones especially close to the brain stem (Møller 1984).

Oral anticonvulsant drugs

Carbamazepine and phenytoin sodium

Patients with central pain which is temporarily relieved by intravenous lignocaine frequently obtain sustained relief with the oral anticonvulsants carbamazepine or phenytoin sodium (Hatangdi et al 1976). Melding & Goodey (1979) studied 125 tinnitus patients for the effects, firstly, of intravenous lignocaine and secondly, of these same two oral anticonvulsants. Of the patients who experienced complete relief with lignocaine, 62% obtained more than 60% relief with carbamazepine. Of the patients who experienced incomplete but better than 60% relief with lignocaine, 52% gained more than 60% relief with carbamazepine. Patients who did not tolerate carbamazepine or developed a rash were treated with phenytoin sodium and obtained a similar incidence but less degree of relief. Because experience of treating central pain with oral anticonvulsants had been disappointing in patients who did not respond to lignocaine, and because the oral anticonvulsant drugs being used were powerful, with troublesome side effects and toxic reactions, they were not recommended to patients whose tinnitus did not respond to lignocaine. Nevertheless, some of these patients had insisted on receiving treatment, but neither Melding & Goodey (1979) nor Goodey (1981) report any patients who responded to oral anticonvulsants after failing to respond to intravenous lignocaine.

Shea & Harell (1978) reported comparable results to Melding & Goodey using carbamazepine but record several patients who benefited from carbamazepine after obtaining only 20% relief from lignocaine. Unlike Melding & Goodey, Shea & Harell did not obtain useful results with phenytoin sodium. Halmos et al (1982) obtained improvement in 52% of patients with phenytoin sodium and only 18% with carbamazepine, and 14% of patients in each group reported that their tinnitus was made worse. There had been no preceding lignocaine test.

Donaldson (1981) in a double-blind trial found no difference between relief from tinnitus obtained by patients with placebo or with carbamazepine. All patients had been tested with lignocaine but were included in the trial irrespective of response, and the dose used was 100 mg twice daily, which was very much smaller than the minimum doses recommended by Melding & Goodey (1979). Marks et al (1981) found no objective change in tinnitus or hearing following a single dose of 200 mg of carbamazepine. Their patients had not been tested with lignocaine and were selected on the basis that tinnitus was non-fluctuant, unilateral, and associated with normal non-fluctuant hearing, a combination of features which Melding et al (1978) considered least likely to respond to lignocaine or anticonvulsants.

Barbiturates and promidone

Amylobarbitone (amobarbital) was reported by Donaldson (1978) as sometimes producing useful relief from tinnitus. Marks et al (1981) recorded no objective improvement from a single dose of 120 mg but the same selection criteria had been used as with carbamazepine. Primidone, which is broken down in the liver into phenobarbitone, and phenobarbitone itself have both been reported by Shea and Emmett (1981) as giving some relief in some patients.

Sodium valproate

Goodey (1981) reported that sodium valproate had been used with 30 patients producing improvements in tinnitus similar to carbamazepine but very much weaker and slower in onset.

Lignocaine analogues

Tocainide (lignocaine amide) is an analogue of lignocaine which can be taken by mouth. It was reported by Emmett and Shea (1980) as offering superior results to other oral anticonvulsants. The subsequent study (Emmett 1981) indicates that tocainide was most consistently effective when given intravenously or in very large doses. Larsson et al (1984) reported two patients with tinnitus effectively suppressed for two years, but reported difficulty in obtaining or maintaining suppression in other patients. Cathcart (1982) found that patients did not obtain significant help from tocainide when it was used in a double-blind trial. However the 26 patients had been included in the trial irrespective of their response to lignocaine and were given tocainide for only one week during the trial, and then only in the relatively small dose of 400 mg three times a day. This small dose had been accepted by her as a trade-off between toxicity and side effects against the possibility of an improved therapeutic response. Concern about toxicity limited the trials of the closely related antirhythmic agent mexiletine (McCormick & Thomas 1981, Kay 1981).

Other drugs

Betahistine is usually thought of as a specific treatment for Ménière's disease. However, it has been recommended in treatment of tinnitus, but found to be of little (Jacobs & Martin 1978) or no (Kay 1981) help in unselected cases. Vasodilators have been claimed to be helpful in combination with antihistamines (Shulman 1981) but not in combination with vitamin A (Brand 1983). Parenteral vitamin A was at one time a common treatment for tinnitus but was then largely discredited (Baron 1951). A variety of vitamins and drugs have been claimed to give relief, including various members of the vitamin B group, curare, Prostigmin, reserpine and various sedatives. Sodium fluoride has been recommended specifically when tinnitus is associated with otosclerosis (Shambaugh 1977). Recently zinc supplements have been suggested (Shambaugh 1981). Sakata et al (1984) were able to ameliorate tinnitus by injection of steroid solution into the middle ear, but obtained no greater response when lignocaine was infused into the middle ear as well.

Ehrenberger and Brix (1983) report long-term suppression of some forms of tinnitus achieved by intravenous infusion of glutamic acid and glutamic acid diethyl ester. Glutamic acid is thought to be, or to enhance, an afferent cochlear nerve transmitter. We have had many patients in whom foods enriched with monosodium glutamate induce or aggravate tinnitus. We have not tested whether tinnitus resulting from glutamate is increased or decreased by intravenous lignocaine.

EFFECTS OF DIET

A wide variety of foods, drinks and drugs can cause or aggravate tinnitus. Where such agents are a frank cause, symptoms are usually bilateral. Tinnitus may be markedly reduced or even abolished by the withdrawal of a particular food, drink or drug from the diet.

Drugs which permanently damage the inner ear or temporarily disturb its function can cause the tinnitus, and so can large doses of the drugs which influence the neural pathways, including the very same anticonvulsant and antidepressant drugs which are sometimes used to treat tinnitus. Drucker (1979) reviewed 108 papers written between 1964 and 1976 in which tinnitus was reported as a side-effect of drug therapy. The British Committee on Safety of Medicines (personal communication, 1985) between 1964 and 1984 had 615 reports of tinnitus attributed to 176 drugs. Most drugs had only one or two notifications and the relationship may often have been coincidental. High incidences of tinnitus were reported with β-adrenergic blocking agents and the antipyretic analgesics aspirin, indomethacin and naproxen. Other drugs which frequently cause reversible tinnitus include quinine, caffeine and antidepressants, anticonvulsants and the antibiotics doxycycline and minocycline. The number of drugs which may occasionally cause tinnitus is so high that every drug a tinnitus patient is taking should be suspected, especially if there is a correlation between onset and fluctuation of the tinnitus and the introduction or dosage change of the drug.

Food can cause or aggravate tinnitus because of natural ingredients or because of the added preservatives, colouring agents, yeasts and monosodium glutamate. The possibility of food intolerance should always be borne in mind but especially suspected in patients with migraine, Ménière's disease, irritable bowel, asthma, eczema or fluctuating bilateral symptoms. In our experience the foods most commonly identified as a cause of tinnitus have been cheese, chocolate and Chinese dinners. The commonest drinks to cause trouble have been coffee, strong tea, tonic water, red wine and grain-based spirits. In our opinion every patient with tinnitus should have a trial period without coffee, tea or other caffeine-containing drinks. Other dietary agents which are causing or aggravating tinnitus may be exposed by simple dietary manipulations and challenges. If simple investigations do not produce a dramatic solution and suspicion of food intolerance remains high then an allergist should be enlisted to supervise systematic elimination diets and challenges.

Excess alcohol can induce tinnitus in almost anyone and some alcoholic drinks in very small amounts can induce it in susceptible patients. However a small proportion of our tinnitus sufferers have reported marked control of their tinnitus when extremely modest amounts of alcohol are used in what has evolved for them into a strict therapeutic regime. Several patients have confided that the onset of their tinnitus followed the use of marijuana. One patient maintains the only way she can get relief from tinnitus is with marijuana. Some patients have admitted to a marked reduction in tinnitus after giving up tobacco smoking.

The extent to which a particular patient finds tinnitus intolerable is not directly related to the loudness of the tinnitus measured objectively. A patient's general, mental and physical health influences the degree to which the tinnitus is noticeable and the degree to which the patient can cope with it. Quite apart from the avoidance of major food intolerances it may well be that a balanced diet, free from excesses, coupled with regular exercise and sensible stress control measures can all contribute to better overall health and less troublesome tinnitus.

LIGNOCAINE TEST

The evidence already presented shows that intravenous lignocaine can dramatically though transiently relieve tinnitus in many patients. It can make some patients worse, and have little effect on others. While intermittent intravenous infusions of lignocaine have been suggested as a treatment protocol, we prefer to regard the use of lignocaine purely as a test to distinguish patients in whom anticonvulsant drugs should be withdrawn from patients who may benefit from the use of anticonvulsant drugs.

Using 1% solution of lignocaine, a maximum dose of 2 mg per kg is drawn into a 20 ml syringe. With the patient lying down, the lignocaine is injected intravenously over two to four minutes whilst pulse rate and patient's reaction to the drug are being monitored. Most patients experience a feeling of fullness in the head, and often slight numbness around the lips. The patient is asked to assess the maximum effect of the lignocaine on their tinnitus. Complete relief is called 100% response, no change 0%, deterioration recorded as worse. Where there is good relief it usually wears off after a few minutes, though occasionally relief has lasted for several days. Once all other subjective effects have worn off the patient is considered safe to drive himself home, usually within half an hour of the injection.

If lignocaine makes tinnitus worse, then any drugs the patient is taking which have an anticonvulsant action are suspect, and we have objective evidence to put before the physician who prescribed them.

If there is little or no improvement with lignocaine, then the chances of improvement with oral anticonvulsants is so small that their use would rarely be justified.

If the response to lignocaine is dramatic, then there is better than 50% chance that large doses of oral anticonvulsant can also achieve useful relief, provided the tinnitus is so bad that the patient is desperate enough to want to take such drugs. On many occasions the positive test result reassures the patient of what can be achieved, and the patient then feels that they can defer the question of drug therapy and cope with their tinnitus after all. In one group of patients about 60% responded both to lignocaine and to the residual inhibition test and the results were cumulative (Goodey 1981). About 20% responded to lignocaine alone, 10% showed residual inhibition alone and 10% responded to neither. This final 10% included a high proportion with near-normal hearing.

ORAL ANTICONVULSANTS AND RELATED DRUGS

The literature already reviewed indicates that the oral anticonvulsant drugs available at present are of no significant help when used in moderate doses for unselected patients who could be helped to tolerate the tinnitus in other ways. Results indicating that oral anticonvulsants have an important role to play have been achieved in patients where tinnitus has been dramatically relieved by lignocaine, but whose tinnitus was so distressing that they were prepared to put up with unpleasant side effects and the risks of toxic reactions in order to achieve a full therapeutic dose. Such patients form only a small proportion of the total group presenting with tinnitus. I suspect many patients have been included in oral anticonvulsant drug trials whose tinnitus could not truly be described as incurable and intolerable, and who should never have been exposed to such powerful drugs. Unless drugs are developed which are specific for the auditory pathways, severe side effects will be inevitable and the use of oral anticonvulsants restricted to patients who are very distressed indeed, who have responded dramatically to the lignocaine test and in whom other methods of treatment have been ineffective.

Carbamazepine (Tegretol®)

This remains the drug of first choice in my opinion. Usually a patient is started on 100 mg (half a tablet) in the evening and the dose is increased by an extra 100 mg daily each week until it reaches 200 mg three times a day. At that stage the white count and serum level are checked and, if necessary, the dose gradually increased again until the tinnitus is tolerable, or further increase in side effects cannot be tolerated, or the maximum therapeutic level of 40 μmol/l is exceeded. In elderly patients we may start with 50 mg at night and increase the dosage even more slowly. In an urgent situation the patient is confined to the house for two weeks and started on the full therapeutic dosage. The most common side effects are drowsiness, forgetfulness and confusion. Where the white count has fallen, the drug dosage has been reduced, and the white count has risen again. If a rash has occurred an antihistamine has been prescribed and carbamazepine withdrawn.

If the maximum dose achieved provides insufficient relief, then a tricyclic is introduced as well (usually nortriptyline 20 mg at night). Once a patient has had time to adjust to the combined drug dosages if the tinnitus is still intolerable and not maskable, then I may gradually introduce phenytoin sodium as well.

If the duration of tinnitus has been relatively short and control with oral drugs is dramatic, then after six months the dosage can be gradually reduced and any return of tinnitus carefully monitored. In most patients we would delay any attempts to wean them off the drugs for one or two years. If reduction in drug dosage is accompanied by increase in tinnitus, patients may remain on oral anticonvulsants indefinitely provided that the white count and serum level are checked every few months. It is unusual to get an adverse reaction after the first six months. Some patients have been disappointed at lack of relief, felt that their tinnitus was not really intolerable and stopped drugs abruptly. After a few days some of these patients have wanted to be put back on the drugs urgently because their tinnitus had returned to what they now recognised as its previous intolerable level.

Phenytoin sodium (Dilantin®)

Phenytoin has proved less effective than carbamazepine and has been used where carbamazepine was withdrawn because of rash, and more recently in combination with carbamazepine and a tricyclic. Previously we avoided using the drugs together because phenytoin is a potent enzyme-inducer and we thought it might interfere with the efficacy of carbamazepine. Experience with central pain indicated their actions were synergic, and we have confirmed this.

Phenytoin is convenient to use, commencing with a paediatric 30 mg capsule three times a day and as the dose is built up changing over to the adult 100 mg capsules and checking the serum level when a full daily dose of 400 mg is reached. Occasionally phenytoin has to be withdrawn because of a rash, but less frequently than with carbamazepine.

Lignocaine amide (Tocainide®)

This is the drug perferred by Emmett & Shea (1980). We have used it effectively in a few patients who got inadequate relief from phenytoin and were too disorientated on carbamazepine. We started with 400 mg at night, gradually increasing the dose over some two months to 600 mg four or five times daily. Recently, great caution has been advised in its use, due to the occurrence of blood dyscrasias.

Sodium valproate (Epilim®, Ergenyl® and Depakine®)

Used in a dose of 200 mg three times a day and 400 mg at night, sodium valproate has a mild ameliorating effect on tinnitus when compared with carbamazepine. Its main use is for patients who have developed a rash with all three of the above drugs.

Antidepressants

Matching tinnitus on a synthesiser shows little correlation between loudness and tolerability. Thus there are two components in the subjective response: the loudness of the tinnitus and the affective reaction to it. Many patients with long-standing hearing loss have abrupt onset of tinnitus associated with a bout of depression or stress. The pattern and frequency of tinnitus corresponds with the hearing loss, suggesting that the affective reaction has altered rather than the basic mechanism. In my experience such patients respond best in the initial instance to antidepressants. Even if the lignocaine test is strongly positive I would advise starting the patient on a tricyclic antidepressant with a relatively small dosage, such as nortriptyline 20 mg at night. Tricyclics have an anticonvulsant as well as antidepressant action and some of these patients claim that their tinnitus is not only more tolerable, but also reduced. As anticonvulsants are subsequently introduced, the dosage required seems to be less or the cumulative effect greater. Where oral anticonvulsant has been introduced in the first place, the subsequent addition of a tricyclic seems to potentiate its action.

Tranquillizers

Benzodiazepines (diazepam, clonazepam) have probably been the most widely prescribed drugs for tinnitus or more particularly for the anxiety associated with it. They do have slight anticonvulsant action and could be helpful in patients who respond to lignocaine, though this has not been demonstrated. These drugs have proved disappointing in the treatment of pain of central origin. They can make a depressed patient worse and could carry a significant risk in a depressed patient whose tinnitus is made worse by lignocaine, as benzodiazepines could aggravate both tinnitus and the associated depression.

Phenothiazines have strong anticonvulsant action, are less depressing than benzodiazepines, and are probably more appropriate for treating anxiety states associated with tinnitus, provided that tinnitus is not aggravated in the lignocaine test. Phenothiazines are sometimes prescribed in combination with tricyclics.

MEDICAL MANAGEMENT OF THE TINNITUS PATIENT

In reviewing the various forms of drug therapy which have been or are being used in the management of tinnitus I have regarded tinnitus as a symptom for which there must be multiple causes and mechanisms. The varied responses to lignocaine appear to justify this assumption. It is quite common for authors to state the same assumption and then to assess individual drugs or therapeutic regimes in terms of the response of unselected groups of patients with tinnitus. From our experience with lignocaine it seems not only unlikely but impossible for any treatment to show up well in such trials. Individual cases which appear to respond to a particular treatment regime need to be analysed, common factors identified, and then controlled trials set up with like groups. As in almost any branch of medicine, logical management of tinnitus boils down to making a diagnosis first, then relating management to that diagnosis and the likely mechanism for the tinnitus associated with it.

The simplest and most common cases of tinnitus

These are patients who appear daily in any otolaryngological practice. The tinnitus is not particularly annoying but the patient is concerned about the possibility of serious implications. Such patients can always be dealt with by the general otolaryngologist and often by a knowledgeable family doctor who has access to modern audiometry. These patients should not need referral to specialised tinnitus or neuro-otological clinics where they may be subjected to investigations out of all proportion to the problem. However, adequate written records should be kept for if the problem needs later reinvestigation early details about the onset have often been forgotten and changes in history, findings and audiometry may be vital.

History

Is tinnitus unilateral or bilateral and if bilateral, is it symmetrical? What is the quality and pitch, is it likened to cicadas, crickets, steam, whistles, bells, a generator, a transformer, the ocean? When did it start and was the onset abrupt or gradual? Does it fluctuate with time of day, mood, foods, drinks, noise? Are there associated symptoms of hearing loss, vertigo, depression, stress, headache, jaw clenching, tooth grinding or stiff neck? What gives relief? What drugs is the patient taking? Does the patient drink excessive amounts of coffee or tea?

Examination

Are there abnormalities of the external or middle ear, nose, nasopharynx, the bite, jaw joints, neck or an auscultation of ear and neck? Is there nearby infection? Does tinnitus persist once wax is removed, infection is controlled or after other simple conditions have been dealt with?

Test for residual inhibition

The correct procedure is described on page 83. Is the tinnitus abolished, reduced or audible only in the other ear? How long is it before the tinnitus returns to its previous level?

Audiometry

Pure tone and speech audiometry and tympanometry are usually sufficient but may need to be repeated when tinnitus is troublesome. Additional tests to distinguish neural from cochlear lesions are reserved for appropriate cases, especially where there is an unexplained asymmetry.

Counselling

In most cases which persist after simple local conditions have been dealt with, the tinnitus corresponds with and can be reasonably attributed to minor inner ear abnormalities which do not in themselves require additional investigation or management. The tinnitus can usefully be explained and understood by the hypothesis that 'lack of stimulus from a damaged part of the inner ear allows over-activity of the corresponding but healthy higher nerve pathway, and that the increased activity is interpreted by the brain as a noise. The sensation of noise is therefore worse with stress, drugs and foods which increase excitability, and is less when plenty of external sound has been transmitted, as confirmed by the crude test of residual inhibition, and the patient's own experiences of masking by environmental sound'.

The patient is reassured that the tests have shown a simple explanation and no evidence of serious disease. The patient is counselled to avoid unnecessary acoustic or other trauma to the ear and to check the extent to which a reduction in stress, caffeine and quinine and any other suspect foods, drinks or drugs may result in a reduction in the intensity of the tinnitus. Simple masking using environmental sound, radios and tape recorders is mentioned, together with the availability of masking devices and powerful drugs for more troublesome cases.

This understanding and reassurance is all that most patients will ever require. *Reassurance without explanation and understanding is seldom sufficient no matter how prestigious the clinician.*

Troublesome cases of tinnitus

Referral to, or further review by, an otolaryngologist becomes necessary if tinnitus remains annoying once any simple conditions about the ear have been dealt with, and if tinnitus continues to increase or is associated with significant deafness, vertigo or ear disease. The otolaryngologist will initially repeat the efforts to recognise and treat any conditions which may be causing or aggravating the tinnitus. Until we have done so, it is premature even to consider the place of powerful drug suppression or time-consuming masking trials.

History

At this stage a questionnaire (Appendix 10.1) will ensure that relevant features are checked for and documented. It is particularly important to note injuries, illnesses and drugs associated with the onset, deterioration or fluctuation of tinnitus. Confirmation of depressive illness, anxiety states, tooth grinding and tooth clenching often require extra interrogation.

Examination and audiometry

A careful comparison is made with the results of any earlier examination and audiometry. Haematological abnormalities, hypothyroidism, hyperthyroidism, syphilis and diabetes are excluded by blood tests. Where appropriate, the clinician should be prepared to test the effects on tinnitus of inserting a grommet, closing a perforation with a rice-paper patch, restricting neck movement with a cervical collar, relaxing the jaw with a temporary dental appliance, excluding possible food allergens with a very restricted diet, and withdrawing suspect drugs. Especially where symptoms are asymmetrical, additional audiological and radiological investigations may be necessary to exclude acoustic neuroma or pressure on the auditory nerve by micro-vascular loops (Møller 1984).

Specific treatments

It is surprising how often a potentially treatable cause or aggravating factor can be initially overlooked. Drugs may be withdrawn, food allergens eliminated, diabetes, thyroid or haematological disorders controlled, wax removed, otitis externa suppressed, Eustachian tube dysfunction compensated for, otosclerosis stabilised with fluoride, glomus tumour removed, conductive hearing loss corrected, Ménière's disease controlled, acoustic neuroma removed or auditory nerve freed from distorting adhesions. Additional noise exposure should be prevented.

Muscle spasm associated with temporomandibular joint dysfunction may be relieved by drug therapy or the jaws may be stabilised with better dentures or a dental appliance. Symptoms aggravated by the neck may respond to manipulation, physiotherapy or the gentle alternative of regular swimming with the patient using the crawl stroke, and breathing on alterate sides.

Of greatest urgency however is the recognition of depression, establishing a positive rapport with a patient who may well be literally at the end of his or her tether and in such cases starting appropriate antidepressant treatment. An attempt to transfer a patient with severe tinnitus to psychiatric care without the otolaryngologist maintaining a positive involvement can be sufficient to trigger a determined suicidal bid.

Counselling

Even a patient whose tinnitus had seemed intolerable and who had required re-assessment may now be reassured by the results of this further examination and investigation together with re-explanation, as already outlined. Simple measures may now be considered adequate and the tinnitus no longer seems sufficiently troublesome to justify the inconveniences of drugs and the expenses of masker trials.

Tinnitus suppression

Test for residual inhibition masking. Patients who have not already been tested for masking potential and residual inhibition are now tested as a prelude to probable aid and/or masker trials. In this context audiological masking with a tinnitus synthesiser is preferred to the crude test described earlier though the results correlate well.

If there is marked and prolonged residual inhibition the audiologist proceeds to fitting of masker and/or aid, depending on the hearing. Tinnitus is subsequently reviewed and a lignocaine test arranged if relief has proved insufficient.

If masking noise is well tolerated but there is little or no residual inhibition then the lignocaine test is arranged (after fitting of an aid if one is needed).

If masking noise is not tolerated then the lignocaine test is arranged and the question of an aid deferred even if one will eventually be needed.

Lignocaine test and anticonvulsant therapy. The lignocaine test (see earlier) is administered to patients selected as described above, following tests for residual inhibition and masking. It is also administered to patients for whom there has been reluctance to withdraw drugs which may already be influencing their tinnitus. The lignocaine test is not usually carried out before the masking trial as the drug would not be needed at all for patients who are easily masked and because it is sometimes followed by such a prolonged response that the tests of residual inhibition and masking would have to be deferred to another day. If masking and/or aids have already been fitted, I prefer the patients to remove these for the lignocaine test as the cumulative effect may give a falsely optimistic response.

If tinnitus is made worse by lignocaine, then it is reasonable to presume that any other drugs with anticonvulsant action will also be aggravating it. We should reconsider non-cochlear causes and modify our explanation to the patient on the basis that there is lower than normal activity, and that the drugs the patient has heard about are contra-indicated. Masking and aiding can still be effective and should be reviewed with increased dedication.

If tinnitus is not greatly altered then anticonvulsant therapy for tinnitus is seldom justified and again the use of aids and masking should be reviewed.

If tinnitus is dramatically relieved then the patient is told that this confirms the original explanation of hyperactivity and that there is a good chance that oral anticonvulsant drugs could achieve a similar though less marked effect. However the patient is warned that a drug which reduces unwanted messages in the hearing nerve pathways will affect other nerve pathways and have unwanted side effects. Many patients, once reassured at what might be achieved, choose to defer the question of oral drug therapy. Others remain desperate and oral treatment is commenced.

I usually start with carbamazepine at night and increase the dose gradually as described earlier until the tinnitus is reduced to a tolerable level, increased side effects cannot be tolerated, or a full therapeutic dose has been achieved. The serum level and white cell count are checked. If the therapeutic or maximum tolerable dose has been reached and relief is insufficient, I add a small dose of trycyclic (usually nortriptyline 20 mg at night). If mild depression has been considered a factor, the tricyclic is introduced before carbamazepine. If relief is still inadequate, I add phenytoin as well. If a rash occurs or carbamazepine is withdrawn for other reasons and the patient remains desperate, then I replace the carbamazepine with either phenytoin or occasionally tocainide. If none of these are tolerated or all three cause a rash, then sodium valproate may still be tolerated though the effect on tinnitus is weaker.

Once a stable drug regime is established, the tolerance of aids and/or maskers may have improved and can be reviewed if the tinnitus is still unacceptable.

Biofeedback

If responses to both residual inhibition test and lignocaine test were disappointing or susbequent trials of maskers and/or drugs were ineffective or abandoned, then biofeedback is considered, provided the patient seems able to co-operate and a programme is available close to their home. Biofeedback is also considered as a specific treatment where stress has been recognised as a major factor often associated with bruxism.

Recalcitrant cases

There remains a residual group of patients for whom everything has failed. I advise against labyrinthectomy or nerve section. I explain that we cannot yet predict the occasional patient who may benefit, that tinnitus may be made worse, and that a main route for later treatments with electrical stimulators or cochlear implants would be destroyed. Voluntary support groups are strongly recommended. The clinician must be prepared to review the patients at intervals to help them to continue to cope with their problem knowing that they have not been abandoned.

REFERENCES

Barany R 1936 Die Beeinflussung des Ohrensausens durch intravenös injizierte Lokalanästhetica. Acta Otolaryngologica 23: 201–203

Baron S 1951 Experiences with parenteral vitamin A therapy in deafness and tinnitus. Laryngoscope 61: 530–547

Brand H 1983 Neural therapy in tinnitus. Wiener Medizinische Wochenschrift 133: 545–547

Cathcart J M 1982 Assessment of the value of tocainide hydrochloride in the treatment of tinnitus. Journal of Laryngology and Otology 96: 981–984

Causse J B, Causse J R, Bel J et al 1984 Result and treatment of tinnitus in our clinic. Annales d'Otolaryngologie et Chirurgie Cervicofaciale 101: 231–235

Donaldson I 1978 Tinnitus: a theoretical view and a therapeutic study using amylobarbitone. Journal of Laryngology 92: 123–130

Donaldson I 1981 Tegretol: a double blind trial in tinnitus. Journal of Laryngology 95: 947–951

Drucker T 1979 Drugs that can cause tinnitus. American Tinnitus Association Newsletter 4(1): 3–5

Duckert L G, Rees T S 1983 Treatment of tinnitus with intravenous lidocaine, a double-blind randomized trial. Otolaryngology and Head and Neck Surgery 91: 550–555

Ehrenberger K, Brix R 1983 Glutamic acid and glutamic acid diethylester in tinnitus treatment. Acta Otolaryngologica 95: 599–605

Emmett J R 1981 Drugs and tinnitus. Discussion. In: Evered D, Lawrenson G (eds) Tinnitus. Ciba Foundation Symposium 85. Pitman, London, pp 275–276

Emmett J R, Shea J J 1980 Treatment of tinnitus with tocainide hydrochloride. Otolaryngology and Head and Neck Surgery 88: 442–446

Englesson S, Larsson B, Lindquist N G, Lyttkens L, and Stahle J 1976 Accumulation of ^{14}C-lidocaine in the inner ear. Acta Otolaryngologica 82: 297–300

Fowler E P Jr 1953 Intravenous procaine in the treatment of Ménière's disease. Annals of Otology Rhinology and Laryngology 62: 1186–1200

Gejrot T 1963 Intravenous xylocaine in the treatment of Ménière's disease. Acta Otolaryngologica Supplement 188: 190

Gejrot T 1976 Intavenous xylocaine in the treatment of attacks of Ménière's disease. Acta Otolaryngologica 82: 301–302

Goodey R J 1981 Drugs in the treatment of tinnitus. In: Evered D, Lawrenson G (eds) Tinnitus. Ciba Foundation Symposium 85. Pitman, London, pp 263–278

Halmos P, Molnar L, Kormos J 1982 Erfahrungen mit Antikonvulsiva bei der Behandlung des Tinnitus. HNO-Praxis 7: 59–61

Hatangdi V S, Boas R A, Richards E G 1976 Post herpetic neuralgia management with antiepileptic and tricyclic drugs. In: Bonica J J, Albe-Fessard D (eds) Advances in pain research and therapy. Proceedings of the First World Congress on Pain, Florence 1975. Raven Press, New York, Vol 1: 583–587

Israel J M, Connelly J S, McTigue S T, Brummett R E, Brown J 1982 Lidocaine in the treatment of tinnitus aurium. A double-blind study. Archives of Otolaryngology 108: 471-473

Jackson P D 1981 Drugs and tinnitus discussion. In: Evered D, Lawrenson G (eds) Tinnitus. Ciba Foundation Symposium 85. Pitman, London, pp 276–278

Jacobs P, Martin G 1978 The therapy of tinnitus resulting from blast injury. HNO 26: 104–106

Kay N J 1981 Oral chemotherapy in tinnitus. British Journal of Audiology 15: 123–124

Larsson B, Lyttkens L, Wäsrteström S A 1984 Tocainide and tinnitus. Clinical effect and site of action. J Otorhinolaryngol Relat Spec 46: 24–33

Lewy R B 1937 Treatment of tinnitus aurium by the intravenous use of local anaesthetic agents. Archives of Otolaryngology 25: 178–183

McCormick M S, Thomas J N 1981 Mexiletine in the relief of tinnitus: a report on a sequential double-blind crossover trial. Clinical Otolaryngology 6: 255–258

Majumdar B, Mason S M, Gibbin K P 1983 An electrocochleographic study of the effects of lignocaine on patients with tinnitus. Clinical Otolaryngology 8: 175–180

Marks N J, Onisiphorou C, Trounce J R 1981 The effect of single doses of amylobarbitone sodium and carbamazepine in tinnitus. Journal of Laryngology and Otology 95: 941–945

Martin F W, Colman B H 1980 Tinnitus: a double-blind crossover controlled trial to evaluate the use of lignocaine. Clinical Otolaryngology 5: 3–11

Melding P S, Goodey R J 1979 The treatment of tinnitus with oral anticonvulsants. Journal of Laryngology and Otology 93: 111–122

Melding P S, Goodey R J, Thorne P R 1978 The use of intravenous lignocaine in the diagnosis and treatment of tinnitus. Journal of Laryngology and Otology 92: 115–121

Møller A R 1984 Pathophysiology of tinnitus. Annals of Otology Rhinology and Laryngology 93: 39–44

Sakata E, Nakazawa H, Iwashita N 1984 Therapy of tinnitus. Tympanic cavity infusion of lidocaine and steroid solution. Auris Nasus Larynx 11: 11–18

Shambaugh G E 1977 Further experiences with moderate dosage sodium fluoride for sensorineural hearing loss, tinnitus and vertigo due to otospongiosis. Advances in Otorhinolaryngology 22: 35–42

Shambaugh G E 1981 Medical management of sensorineural losses: Inner ear problems. Ear Clinics International 1: 65–70

Shea J J, Emmett J R 1981 The medical treatment of tinnitus. Journal of Laryngology and Otology (Supplement 4): 130–138

Shea J J, Harell M 1978 Management of tinnitus aurium with lidocaine and carbamazepine. Laryngoscope 88: 1477–1484

Shea J J, Emmett J R, Orchik D J, Mays K, Webb W 1981 Medical treatment of tinnitus. Annals of Otology Rhinology and Laryngology 90: 601–609

Shulman A 1981 Vasodilator-antihistamine therapy and tinnitus control. Journal of Laryngology and Otology (Supplement 4): 123–129

TINNITUS STUDY

CHART 1

Family Name	Given Name	Age	Sex
Address		Telephone No.	
Occupation	Referring Specialist		G.P.

	MEDICAL HISTORY	Yes	No	
CVS	Heart Disease			
	Coronory Thrombosis			
	High Blood Pressure			
	Strokes			
R.S.	Bronchitis			
	Emphysema			
	Operations			
	Other			
IMMUNE.	Anaemia			
	Bleeding disorders			
	Rheumatoid Arthritis			
	Other			
ALLERGY	Food			
	Drug			
	Asthma			
	Eczema			
	Hay Fever			
	Other			
RENAL	Kidney disease			
METABOLIC	Diabetes Mellitus			
	Thyroid Disease			
	Pagets disease			
	Hyperlipidaemia			
	Other			
CNS.	Shingles			
	Neuralgia			
	Other			
INFECTIVE	Tuberculosis			
	Mumps			
	Glandular Fever			
	Measles			
	Chicken Pox			
	Other			
TOXIC	Alcohol			
	Tobacco			

Drugs	Gentamycin	Streptomycin	Kanamycin	Neomycin	Other
	Penicillin	Aspirin	Quinine	Diuretics	Other

CURRENT MEDICATION

TINNITUS STUDY **E.N.T. ASSESSMENT** **CHART 2**

NAME   AGE

TINNITUS	side	right		left	
	duration				
	pitch	high / low		high / low	
	quality	continuous / pulsatile		continuous / pulsatile	
	pattern	steady / fluctuating		steady / fluctuating	
		silence		silence	
		noise		noise	
		fatigue		fatigue	
		tension		tension	
		cold		cold	
		alcohol		alcohol	
		tobacco		tobacco	
		hypnagogic		hypnagogic	
		other		other	
HEARING LOSS		right		left	
	none / slight / moderate / severe			none / slight / moderate / severe	
		stable / fluctuating		stable / fluctuating	
		silence		silence	
		noise		noise	
		fatigue		fatigue	
		tension		tension	
		cold		cold	
		alcohol		alcohol	
		tobacco		tobacco	
		other		other	
UNSTEADINESS	nil		constant	fluctuating	

		When	How Long	Quality	Other features
	previous				
VERTIGO	episodic				
	positional				
	postural				

EAR DISCHARGE		right	left	
EARACHE		right	left	
EAR OPERATIONS	what	right	left	
	when			

TINNITUS STUDY

CHART 2 (cont'd)

ASSOCIATED SYMPTOMS

		right	left	
NOSE	blockage			
	discharge			
	P.N.D.			
	sneezing			
JAW	pain			
	clicking			
NECK	pain			
	stiffness			
	whiplash			
HEADACHE				
HEAD INJURY				
FAMILY HISTORY	tinnitus			
	hearing loss			
	dizzy attacks			
	ear disease			
	ear operations			

TINNITUS STUDY   **CHART 4**

NAME .... AGE ....

I.V. LIGNOCAINE TEST

Date .... Patient's weight .... Dose ....

Results:

	V.A. % Relief
TINNITUS	100%
	Over 60%
	30 – 60%
	Less than 30%
	No change
	Increase
DEAFNESS	Much better
	Moderately better
	Slightly better
	No change
	Slightly worse
	Moderately worse
	Much worse

Comments:

11   *J. W. P. Hazell*

Guidelines for the Management of Tinnitus

1. Identification and treatment of underlying causes

   a. In the ear
      - (i) wax
      - (ii) conductive hearing loss
      - (iii) other conditions amenable to treatment, e.g. Ménière's disease/cochlear otosclerosis
   b. Systemic
      - (i) drugs: adverse effects of
      - (ii) food allergy
      - (iii) dental malocclusion/TMJ disorders
      - (iv) hypertension
      - (v) anaemia/dyslipidaemia
      - (vi) hypothyroidism
      - (vii) diabetes
      - (viii) syphilis
      - (ix) hypoglycaemia (especially early morning)
      - (x) cervical disorders
   c. Early acoustic neuroma. All unilateral tinnitus should be investigated (e.g. BSER/radiography).

2. Explanation of the mechanism of tinnitus

Reassurance and prognosis
Review of treatment options
Stress that tinnitus does not mean cancer/imminent stroke/psychiatric condition

   No treatment needed for
   a. Very short duration tonal tinnitus ('physiological')
   b. Very quiet continuous tinnitus not causing distress and masked by any environmental sound
   c. Tinnitus following noise exposure (but hearing conservation advice must be given)

3. **Palliation by prosthetic management (maskers etc.)**
    a. Any hearing disability (of which the patient may not be aware)—consider amplification
    b. No demonstrable communication difficulties (or hearing aid giving insufficient help with tinnitus)—trial of masking device or devices, combination hearing aid/masker, parallel hearing aid(s) and masker fittings
    c. Initial failure of prosthetic management—check:
        Have all permutations been tried, including binaural fittings?
        Is ear canal inappropriately occluded?
        Has proper counselling and instruction been given?

4. **Psychological/psychiatric management**
    a. If depression/anxiety a worse problem than tinnitus, consider anti-depressants, appropriate referral, but avoid dependency-creating drugs and prolonged therapy.
    b. If tinnitus is promoting or creating anxiety
        relaxation techniques
        behaviourable psychology
        instructional tapes/literature (these are a valuable adjunct to all therapy)
    c. Appropriate management of sleep disturbance
    d. Membership of self-help or patient support group e.g. local tinnitus groups, national tinnitus associations*, use of lay counsellors (who may be tinnitus patients)

5. **Where these approaches fail: consider**
    a. Drug therapy ('membrane stabilizers', anti-epileptics (see Chapter 10))
        (i) occasional long-term responders occur
        (ii) this may be only option with tinnitus in a dead ear
    b. Chronic electrical stimulation with implanted electrode (see Chapter 6).
    c. Sympathetic view of patients' ideas about alternative medicine

*American Tinnitus Association
 PO Box 5
 Portland, Oregon 97207
 USA
 Telephone (503) 248-9985

*British Tinnitus Association
 105 Gower Street
 London WC1E 6AH
 Telephone (01) 387-8033

Author Index

Adams F. 5
Aitken L. M. 30
Alexander of Trailles 4, 5
Alpers B. J. 135
Altmann 74, 150
American Tinnitus Association 72
Anderson S. D. 34, 148
Angelicus 1
Anglicus 5
Anon 1, 58
Appelbaum F. L. 147
Aran J-M. 118
Arenberg I. K. 146
Aristotle 4, 71, 96
Arlen H. 149
Armstrong-Bednall G. 56
Asherson N. 8
Ashley J. 71
Avicenna 5

Babin R. 149
Bacon F. 1, 6
Baker L. J. 161, 165, 166
Barany R. 176
Baron S. 179
Bartel M. 1
Békésy G. von 21, 22, 23
Bergman M. 104, 157
Berliner K. I. 119
Bernstein J. M. 39, 149
Bertrand R. A. 147
Blair Simmons F. 150
Bolland J. J. 6, 7
Boulet J. J. 146
Brackmann D. E. 118, 151, 152
Brand H. 179
Brenner R. 9, 13
Bretlau P. 150
British Committee on Safety of Medicines 180
Brix 179
Brown A. M. 36
Brown J. 137
Brown R. D. 15
Brownell W. E. 28, 37

Browning G. G. 59
Burns V. 24
Butler J. 134, 137, 139

Campbell Thomson R. 2
Capranica R. R. 37
Carey F. H. 146
Carmody R. F. 147
Cartheuser J. F. 6, 9
Cathcart, J. M. 179
Causse J. B. 150, 177
Causse J. R. 108
Cazals Y. 27, 118
Celsus 4
Chambers C. 162
Chandler J. R. 146
Charissoux G. 150
Chouard C-H. 118, 169
Chum R. 34, 35
Clark W. W. 35, 36, 37
Coles R. R. A. 46, 49, 50, 52, 53, 56, 57, 59,
    71, 131, 134, 157, 161, 164, 173
Colman B. H. 177
Conrad-Armes D. 38, 58, 84, 163
Corcoran A. 159
Costen J. B. 149
Crasius 6
Crawford A. C. 28
Crisp A. H. 164
Crown S. 164

Dallos P. 26, 27, 39
Dandy, W. E. 151
Danley M. J. 120
Darwin E. 9
Davis A. C. 26, 50, 52, 53, 56
Davis H. 77
de Boer E. 24
de Chauliac G. 5
de Gordon B. 5
Donaldson I. 178
Douek E. 97, 150
Drucker T. 180

197

Du Verney J. G. 1, 8
Duckert L. G. 177

Ehrenberger K. 179
Elberling C. 34
Elliott E. 34
Emmett J. R. 133, 177, 178, 179
Empedocles 3
Englesson S. 176
Epley J. M. 147
Erlandson S. 170
Ersner M. S. 17, 96
Evans E. F. 24, 29, 34, 36, 37, 39, 41
Evered D. 58

Fallopius G. 6
Feldmann H. 9, 39, 82, 105, 106
Fenwick J. A. 118
Fernelius J. 6
Fettiplace R. 28
Finckenau J. 6
Fisch U. 152
Fleminger J. J. 58
Flock A. 96
Flood L. M. 151
Forster E. S. 5, 96
Fowler E. P. 17, 73, 74, 78, 79, 162, 173, 176
Fraysse B. 152
Fretz R. J. 120
Freud C. 138

Galen 4
Gallet J. 148
Garrison F. H. 9
Gejrot T. 176
Gelb H. 149
George B. 146
Gibson R. 145
Glanville J. D. 22, 35, 131
Glasgold A. 74, 150
Glasscock M. E. 152
Gold T. 25, 33, 38
Goodey R. J. 80, 133, 177, 178, 179, 181
Goodhill V. 73, 150
Goodwin P. E. 9, 78, 80, 162
Graham J. T. 73, 118, 132, 134, 135, 137, 139
Grapengeisser C. J. C. 9, 118
Greist S. 74
Grossan M. 169, 170, 171
Guerrier Y. 1
Guirand F. 3
Guthrie D. 18

Haggard M. P. 56
Hallam R. S. 58, 159, 161, 162, 163, 164, 165, 166, 168, 172, 173
Halmos P. 178
Halstead T. H. 148
Hansen P. E. 170
Harrell M. 177, 178

Harris D. 39
Harris S. 106, 146
Harrison 40
Harrison R. V. 41
Hartmann M. 6, 7
Hatangdi V. S. 176, 178
Hatton D. S. 118
Hazell J. W. P. 54, 55, 57, 58, 73, 78, 99, 101, 102, 104, 105, 106, 107, 108, 109, 110, 113, 114, 118, 134, 138, 145, 149, 150, 162, 163, 164
Heller M. F. 104, 157
Hinchcliffe R. 49, 53, 157, 161, 162, 165
Holgate R. C. 145
House W. 118, 119, 128, 129, 151, 152, 158, 164
House P. R. 170, 171

Institute of Hearing Research 46, 48, 50, 57, 101, 104
Illum P. 135
Israel J. M. 80, 177
Itard J. M. C. 9, 11, 17, 96
Ito K. 147

Jackson P. 148, 152, 177
Jacobs P. 179
Jakes S. C. 163, 166, 167, 172, 173
Jakimetz J. R. 52
Jannetta P. J. 147
John of Gaddesden 6
Johnsen N. J. 34
Johnson R. M. 78, 80, 109, 157, 162
Johnstone B. M. 24, 26, 96
Jones I. H. 17, 96, 106

Kamal H. 2
Kay N. J. 179
Kemp D. T. 25, 33, 34, 35, 36, 38, 96, 133
Kennedy 170
Khanna S. M. 21, 25
Kiang N. Y. S. 24, 29, 39
Kim D. O. 36
King-Hele D. 9
Klinke R. 37
Klochoff I. 22, 148, 149
Knudsen V. O. 17, 96
Kudo T. 147
Kuhn C. G. 4

Lackner J. R. 77
Lane H. 9
Larsson B. 179
Lawrenson G. 58
Lazorthes Y. 152
Leca A-P. 2
Lempert J. 149
Leonard D. G. B. 25
Leschevin 9

Leske M. C. 49, 52
Leveque H. 147
Lewy R. B. 80, 176
LeZak M. H. V. 133, 134
Liberman M. C. 30, 39
Liedenfrost J. G. 6
Littre E. 4
Lusk R. 149
Lyndberg P. 171
Lyttkens D. J. 41

MacKinnon D. M. 138, 149
Macleod-Morgan C. 171
MacNaughton-Jones H. 13
Maillard C. 15
Majumdar B. 177
Malatesta V. J. 170
Manley G. A. 30, 34, 36
Marchiando A. 148
Marks N. J. 170, 178
Marlowe F. I. 171
Martin F. W. 146, 177, 179
Martin M. C. 99
McCormick M. S. 179
McCreary H. S. 146
McFadden D. 34, 39, 102, 158, 162, 163, 169
Meador K. J. 146
Meikle M. B. 54, 57, 74, 76, 78, 79, 81, 83, 105
Melding P. S. 80, 176, 177, 178
Mendel D. 98
Merluzzi F. 56
Mesue 5
Michelangelo 71
Miller M. H. 52
Mitchell C. 162
Moffat A. J. M. 37
Moller A. R. 32, 98, 177, 186
Mollestrom A. R. 106
Mongan E. 39
Muller J. 12
Myers E. N. 39

National Center for Health Statistics 71
Newton T. H. 146
Nodar R. H. 131, 133, 134
Nunley J. 99

O'Connor A. F. 23, 147
Office of Population Censuses and Surveys 49, 52, 104, 162
Ogawera S. et al 147
Ogden M. S. 5
Opsomer-Halleux C. 5

Palmer A. R. 37
Paracelsus 6
Paul of Aegina 5
Pederson C. B. 151
Penner M. J. 39, 81, 162

Pialoux P. 118
Plattsmier H. S. 34
Pliny 4
Politzer A. 1, 4, 5, 6, 7, 12, 138, 148
Porter W. G. 17
Portmann M. 118
Prijs V. P. 40, 41
Pseudo-Aristotle 5
Pulec J. L. 147, 151

Rabinowitz W. M. 38
Reed G. F. 73, 78, 149, 162, 163
Rees T. S. 177
Reich G. 133, 134, 157
Reid J. 97, 150
Reymond E. A. E. 2
Rhode W. S. 24, 25
Riolan the younger 5, 7
Robertson D. 30
Robinson D. W. 52
Rogers C. R. 113
Rothstein J. 116
Ruggero M. A. 35, 37
Russell I. J. 27

Sakata E. 179
Saltzman M. 17, 96
Salvi R. J. 39
Savary P. 150
Schedel J. H. 6
Schenck J. T. 6
Schleuning A. J. 81, 101, 102, 109
Schloth E. 34, 38
Schmiedt R. A. 39
Schuff N. 74
Schuknecht H. F. 41
Schwartze 147
Scott B. 171, 172
Sellick P. M. 25, 27
Shambaugh G. E. Jr. 108, 179
Shea J. J. 23, 147, 177, 178, 179
Sheldrake J. B. 105, 109, 112
Schulman A. 118, 129, 179
Smolders J. 37
Snashall S. E. 132, 135
Spalding J. A. 17, 73, 75, 82, 151
Spencer W. G. 4
Spitzer J. B. 110
Spoendlin H. 28
Staab W. 99
Stephens S. D. G. 1, 2, 3, 5, 9, 15, 17, 158, 159, 164, 165, 168, 169, 173
Stevenson R. S. 18
Strack G. 36
Stroud M. H. 148
Suga N. 24
Sutton G. J. 22, 34, 35, 52, 149
Sweetow R. W. 173
Swift T. R. 146

Taylor-Walsh E. 57
Terry A. M. P. 106
Tewfik S. 108, 145
Thedinger B. 118, 129
Thomas I. B. 34, 179
Tonndorf J. 21, 38
Toynbee J. 150
Tyler R. S. 38, 58, 84, 161, 163, 165, 166

Valescus of Tranta 5
Vallis R. C. 146
Valvassori G. E. 147
Vernon J. 39, 79, 81, 82, 83, 96, 102, 105, 109, 118, 150, 151
Volta A. 9

Walford R. E. 22, 157
Walsh E. T. 76, 78, 79, 81, 146
Ward P. H. 146
Watanabe I. U. 148, 149

Webster W. R. 30
Wegel R. L. 77
Weiss T. F. 24, 37
Wepfer J. J. 8, 17
Wever E. G. 24
Whitney S. 78
Wibel G. D. 9
Widkin G. P. 38
Wiggers H. C. 148
Wilde W. 13
Wilson H. 17, 96
Wilson J. P. 22, 24, 33, 34, 35, 36, 37, 38, 96, 97, 149
Wood S. M. 105, 106, 109
Wright A. 5

Yanick P. 169

Zeidler 6
Zurek P. M. 34, 35, 36, 37, 38
Zwicker E. 34, 35, 36

Subject Index

Abstinence from alcohol 4
Acouphenes 1
Acoustic nerve section 144, 151, 152, 188
Acoustic neuroma 108, 144, 152
Acoustic trauma 149
Actin 96
Action potential 27
Active mechanical processes 25, 38
Acupuncture, placebo trial 170
Adaptation to tinnitus 101, 159
 see also Habituation 81
Afferent cochlear fibres 28
Age 50
 and gender 53
 and noise, effect on tinnitus 50
 of onset 56
Air trapped in the ear, cause of 6
All-in-the-ear aids 110
Amylobarbitone 178
Anaemia 108
Angiography 145, 146
Animal models of tinnitus 39
Annamites 2
Annoyance of tinnitus 61
 in children 136
 time course 60
Anoxia and tinnitus 74
Anterior inferior cerebellar artery 147
Antibiotics 176
Anticonvulsants 177, 180, 181, 183
Antidepressants 74
Antihistamines 179
Anxiety 113, 165
Arteriopathy 108
Arteriovenous malformations 146–147
Aspirin 39, 180
 avoidance 85
Assessment of tinnitus,
 recommended procedure 75
 analogy with bridge 73
 in children 139
Associated symptoms, importance of 164
Assyrians, views 2
Asthma 180

Asymmetrical tinnitus 112
Auckland pain clinic 176
Audiogram, tinnitus makes it difficult 137
Audiological scientist 103
Audiometric tests, poor predictor 104
Audiometry 47, 185
 descending vs. ascending 137
 repeated 115
Auditory rehabilitation 115
Aural toilet 4
Auscultation—
 ear 147
 head and neck 73
 neck 138

Backlog of patients 57
Balanites oil 2
Basilar membrane—
 mechanics 23
 properties 24
Beats with tinnitus 38, 77
Beethoven 71
Bending down 147
Benzodiazepines 184
Beta blockers 59, 180
Betahistine 179
Bewitchment of ears 2
Bilateral tinnitus 81
Binaural tinnitus 112
Biofeedback 164, 170, 171, 188
Blood flow, cause 21
Blood-letting 11
Blow to the ear 6
Bourdonnements 1
British Tinnitus Association 55
Bruits 145

Caffeine 180
 avoidance 85
Canal aids 110
CAP audiograms 41

201

Carbamazepine   178, 182
    first choice   182
    side effects   182
Cardiovascular disorder   59
Crown-Crisp Experiential Index (CCEI)   164
Central auditory pathways   30
Central control of tinnitus   98
Central fusion of cochlear tinnitus   35
Central pain relieved by anticonvulsants   178
Central tinnitus, models   32
Cervical spine, cause of tinnitus   144
Characteristic frequency   27, 29
Cheese   180
Children   131–155
    prevalance of tinnitus   132
    with spontaneous otoacoustic emissions   35
    tolerance in   131
    type of tinnitus   134
Chinchilla, spontaneous otoacoustic
        emissions   37
Chinese food   180
Chinese torture, analogy   78
Chocolate   180
Classification of patients   157, 164
    by McNaughton-Jones   13
Clenching the teeth   149
Clicking tinnitus   148, 156
Clinical attendance, with age   56
    populations   54
    for tinnitus UCH London   103
Clinical services—
    examination   47
    features   54
    planning   46
Clonazepam   184
Cochlear aqueduct   145
Cochlear implant   120, 188
    and buzzing tinnitus   125
    effects on tinnitus   121, 123
    for tinnitus alone   129
Cochlear implantation   118–130
Cochlear model for tinnitus and masking   96
Cochlear microphonic   27
Cochlear nerve—
    properties   29
    spontaneous activity   29
Cochlear nucleus   30
Cockroaches   4
Cocktail-party effect   21
Coffee   180
Cognitive therapy   173
Coherent masking   82
Cold showers   11
Combination instruments   99, 101, 110
Combined therapy   80, 182
Comfortable listening level   162
Comparative anatomy of ear   24
Complainers   166
Complete residual inhibition   83
Complex tinnitus   78

Compression of auditory nerve   147
Computerized tomography   147
Concentration   71
Concentration loss   165
Conductive deafness   149
Confusion   165
Congenital middle ear abnormalities   135
Continuous masking therapy   106
Contraction of palatine muscles, cause of   12
Contralateral testing   81
Corti, organ of   28
Cortical arousal   161
Coryza, cause of   4
Counselling   113, 164, 185
Crackling   148
Crickets   77
Cry for help   158
CSOM   135
Curare   179
Cystic astroblastoma   146

DC potentials   26
Dead ear tinnitus   112
Deafness   164
Deafness aetiology and tinnitus in children   134
Depakine®   183
Depression   7, 74, 104, 113, 164, 165, 166
Descriptives, need for range of   48
Despair   165
Destructive ear surgery, effect on tinnitus   151
Determinants of tinnitus   50
Device for occluding jugular vein   146
Diabetes   186
Diary keeping   115
Diazepam   184
Diet and tinnitus   7
Dietary trials   180
Digital subtraction angiography   147
Dilantin®   183
Dilatation of blood vessels, cause   12
Disability caused by tinnitus   115
Distress   103, 157, 159, 161, 176
Distress and annoyance   163
    from different causative factors   164
    and loudness of tinnitus not related   156, 162
    and tinnitus loudness   161
Diuretics, loop   59
Dizziness   164
    and tinnitus in children   135
    unrelated to test results   165
Domiciliary visiting, household study   47
Doxycycline   180
Drug dependance   165
Drug therapy   166, 176–190
    dose reduction   182
    a side effect   180

Ear plug effect   8, 21, 110, 149
    plugs   109
    protectors, increased use of   50
    suction   6

Earmould choice for masking 109
 open 110
Eczema 180
Effect of tinnitus on life 48
 with age 56
Effect of media 161
Efferent supply to cochlea 29, 30, 98
Electricity 9
Electrical suppression of tinnitus 13, 27, 152, 169
Electrical stimulation—
 transcutaneous 118
 transtympanic 118
Embolization with gelatine sponge 146
Emotional problems 165
Endolymphatic hydrops 135
 sac 150
Environmental masking 115, 158, 161
Enzymes in otosclerosis 150
Epidemiology of tinnitus 46–70
Epilepsy 135
Epilim® 183
Ergenyl® 183
Ethacrynic acid 34
Eustachian tube 23
 catheterization 9
 cautery 147
 clicks 21
 diathermy 148
 Telfon® injection 148
Evaluation of therapy 169
Examination 185
 importance of 74
Exercise 4
External carotid artery 146
 ear canal 21
 sound different from tinnitus 39, 80
Eyelid blinking and tinnitus 148

Factors relieving tinnitus 123
 affecting tinnitus 122
False tinnitus 10
Famous sufferers 17
Fantastic tinnitus 10
Faradism 13
Fat-wire prostheses 150
Fatigue 123
Fears of malignancy 156
Feebleness of the ears, cause 5
Feldmann masking curves 106
Females, better hearing 53
Fevers 4
Fluoride therapy 150
Follow-up visits 115
Food additives 180
Frankincense 2
Frustration 165
Fullness in ear 147
Fumigation, with snale skin 2
 with aromatic substances 3

Funding for tinnitus research, poor 72
Fusion of tinnitus 112

Galvanic stimulation 118
Galvanism 13
Gargling 4
Gender, determining factor in tinnitus 52
General Household Survey (IHR) 46, 49
General practitioner, when consulted 56
Geographical influences 54
Getting to sleep 165
Glutamic acid (and diethyl ester) 179
Gradual onset tinnitus 60
Greater petrosal sinus 146
Guinea pig, spontaneous otoacoustic emissions 37

Habituation, 61, 81, 159
 see also Adaptation
Haematological investigations 59
 screen 47
Hair cell 96
 resonators 25
 responses 27
Hairs on tympanic membrane 74
Hallucinations, auditory 2
Handedness and tinnitus laterality 57
Head injury 77, 146
Headache 136, 165, 166, 170
Health measures, general 181
Health worries 167
Hearing aids 99, 139
 compression, need in tinnitus 138
 effect on tinnitus 123
 less effective than maskers 110
 setting in children with tinnitus 138
 tinnitus louder after use 106
 use difficult with tinnitus 138
 use in children, provoking tinnitus 134
Hearing deterioration—
 difficulties not related to thresholds 168
 difficulties vs. tinnitus distress 104
 difficulty independent of tinnitus 166
 loss and tinnitus 81, 110, 104, 164
 masked by tinnitus (Celsus) 4
 prevention 151
 professionals, training 158
 thresholds, deaf children 132
Hereditary disposition, cause 7
Hissing tinnitus 78
History taking 103, 184
Holistic approach 7, 83, 114
Horseradish peroxidase 30
House Ear Institute 118
Humours 3, 5
Hums 22
Hydrocephalus 146
Hyperacusis 109
Hypnosis 171
Hypochondriasis 11, 157
Hypoxia 34

Idiopathic tinnitus 144
Immunological disorders 176
In-the-head tinnitus 112
Incidence *see* Prevalence
Incongruous sound 156
Incudo-stapedial joint, subluxation 148
Indomethacin 180
Inner ear, function 23
Innervation of hair cells 28
Insomnia 173
Interference with life 120, 126
Intermittent vs. constant tinnitus 134
Interpretation of cause of tinnitus 156
Intracranial hypertension 145
Intra-meatal microphone 108
Intratympanic muscles 148
Intrusiveness of tinnitus 166
Irregular vascular lumen 145
Irritable bowel syndrome 180
Irritant footbaths 11
Irritation 165

Jaw movement, cause of tinnitus 22
Jugular bulb, asymmetry 146

Kemp echo 22, 23, 34

Labyrinthectomy 144, 151, 188
Lateral sinus–jugular vein anastomosis 146
'Learning to live with tinnitus' 61
Leeches 11, 13
Left ear predominance of tinnitus? 57
Lidocaine, *see* Lignocaine
Life-style changes 165
Ligation of jugular vein 146
Lignocaine 40, 80, 152, 176, 183
  analogues 179
  effective in periphery 177
  test in cochlear neurectomy selection 152
Localized to the head, masking of tinnitus 82
Locating sound 20
Location of tinnitus 73
Loop diuretics 59
Lorcainide and sleep disturbance 177
Loud sounds, avoidance of 85
Loudness, of tinnitus 58, 123, 125
  discomfort levels 84
  and distress 163
  and intrusiveness 168
  matching 78, 162, 163, 172
  measures of tinnitus considering recruitment 84
  rating of tinnitus 120
  of tinnitus, time course 60
  variations of tinnitus 163
Low-pitched tinnitus 150
Lumbar puncture 146

Marijuana 85, 180
Maskability of tinnitus 162

Maskers 96, 99
  body-worn 99
  first fitting 112
  fitting 109, 110
  high powered 110
  at night 115
  programmable 106
  reliability 101
  usage 115
Masking 10, 96, 139, 151, 159, 187
  continuous, best stimulus 106
  contralateral 98, 112
  effect of aids in chldren 134
  effect on cochlear 98
  effect on hearing 114
  and electrical suppression, relationship 129
  by environmental noise 11
  by environmental sounds 5
  first harmonic generator 17
  helps sleep 12
  improvement of loudness discomfort 109
  in Ménière's disease 109, 151
  night use 104
  principles 114
  programme 115
  sensation level 112
  sounds 80, 101
  by telephone 17
  therapeutic trial 107
  therapy 96–117
  reasons for failure 110
  tinnitus 'break-through' 112
  with two pebbles 9
  unsuitable for 101
  which ear? 112
  by water-mill 11
Massage 4, 15
Measurements of tinnitus 58
Media, effect of 161
Medical management 184
Membrane stabiliser 177
Ménière's disease 15, 108, 144, 150, 151, 176, 180
  'burnt-out' 150
Meningeal vessels 145, 146
Menstruation 4
Mercury inhalations 5
Middle ear, function 21
  muscles 12
Migraine 180
Mild tinnitus 72
Mineral deficiencies 176
Minimal masking level 80, 112, 162
Minocycline 180
Model for tinnitus—
  cochlear 96
  retrocochlear 98
  tolerance 159
Mondini deformity 135

Monosodium glutamate, aggravating tinnitus 179
Mossbauer technique 24
Multidimensional complaints, factor analysis 166
Mustard in beer 3
Myocin 96
Myoclonus 148
Myringoplasty 149
Myringotomy 13

Naproxen® 180
National Study of Hearing, UK 46
Natural history of tinnitus 60
Nerve section, *see* Acoustic or vestibular nerve section
Nervousness 123
Neural tinnitus due to 'cross-talk' 32
Neuro-otology clinic, unsuitable 173
Noise 50, 51
  exposure, cause 50
  exposure and tinnitus laterality 58
Noise-induced hearing loss 149
Noise-induced short-duration tinnitus 6
'Non-clinical' tinnitus 50
Non-complaining subjects 163
Normal hearing and tinnitus, most disturbed group 157
Nortriptyline 182, 183
Noticing tinnitus 156
Nottingham Tinnitus Clinic 55
Number and types of tinnitus 125

'Objective' and 'subjective' tinnitus 73
Objective tinnitus 131
  measurements 108
Occlusion effect 21
  see also Ear plug effect
Octave confusion in pitch matching 75
Olivo-cochlear bundle 30
Opium 4
Ossicles, function 21
Otitis, incidence of 149
Otoacoustic emissions 21, 22, 33, 35, 37, 38, 96
  in the Caiman alligator 36
Otolaryngologist, role of 74
Otosclerosis and tinnitus 22, 179
  cochlear 108
  incidence 149
  surgery and tinnitus 150
Ototoxic drugs 15, 180
Outer hair cells, active mechanism 26
Overstimulation of auditory nerve 12

Paget's disease 145, 176
Pain 165, 166
Palatal myoclonus 74, 138, 148
  muscles 12
Papyrus, Egyptian 2

Partial residual inhibition 83
Partially hearing units 131
Patch test 150, 186
Pathological correlates 59
Patulous Eustachian tube 23, 147
Perforation of tympanic membrane 149
Perilymph fistula 135, 150
  test for 151
Personality types noticing tinnitus 158
Personal loudness units 162
Phase locking 29, 30
Phenobarbitone 178
Phenothiazines 184
Phenytion sodium 178, 182, 183
Phobic anxiety 165
Physiological body sounds 157
Pinna 20
Pitch and loudness scaling, correlations 58
  and loudness of tinnitus, confusion 75
  matching 75, 76
  scaling 58
Placebo masking trial 170
  effects 169
Plasma viscosity 59
Positive feedback 25
Postal questionnaires 46
Prevalence of tinnitus 47, 49
  in children 131
    PHU vs. school for deaf
  in USA 71
Primidone 178
Problems created by tinnitus 165
Profound deafness, quality of tinnitus 122
Prognosis of tinnitus 60
Prognostic indicators, tinnitus with implant 127
Prostigmin 179
Pseudo tumor cerebri 146
Psychiatric referral 113
Psychological model for tinnitus 159
  approaches to management 169
  factors 156
Pterygoid muscles 149
Pulsatile tinnitus 22, 145, 146
  treatment by embolization 146
Pulsation of cranial blood vessels 4
Purging 3, 5
Purging avoidance 4

Questionnaire 66, 74, 88, 129, 164, 191
Quinine 180

Raised intracranial pressure 146
Rash 183
Rational view 159
Reassurance 113, 115, 159
Recalcitrant cases 188
Recent-onset cases 169
Recreational activity, effect of tinnitus 104

Recruitment 84, 109, 136
    effect on tinnitus 80
    helped by masking 109
Red wine 180
Relaxation 170
    difficulty 165
    training 170
    using tinnitus as cue 171
Renovaine injection into meatus 177
Reserpine 179
Residual inhibition 82, 105, 114, 138, 185, 187
    best stimulus 106
    explanation of 98
    with implant 129
    not with hearing aids 106
    optimal stimulus 106
    partial 105
    test 105
    test format 83
    total or complete 83, 105
Residual hearing, conservation 144
Respiration, tinnitus in time with 147
Retirement and tinnitus 161
Roaring tinnitus 147
Rustling 148

Salerno, school of 96
Salicylates 34
Scaling of tinnitus 78
Schools for hearing-impaired children 131
'Second filter' 24
Secretory otitis media and tinnitus 134
Sedatives 179
Selection of patients, for masking 101
Self-help groups 166
Sensation level (loudness match) 58
Sensorineural deafness 150
Severe annoyance from tinnitus 50
Severe effect on life 50
Severe tinnitus 49
    incidence 49
    in USA 72
Severity of tinnitus related to hearing loss 53
Sex, abstinence 7
Short duration tinnitus 50
Shunt, subarachnoid–peritoneal 146
Significance of tinnitus 159
Site of tinnitus 57
Sleep—
    disturbance 11, 48, 50, 71, 104, 164, 167
    and gender 52
    getting off to 165, 166
    time course 60
Smetana, Bedrich 71
Smoking 180
Social noise exposure 51
Socio-economic status 54
    and age 55
Sodium fluoride 108, 179
Sodium valproate 179, 183

Somatic anxiety 165
Somatising 157
Spa 15
Specific treatment 186
Spirits, grain based 180
Spontaneous otoacoustic emissions 35, 96
    cause 21, 35
    in dogs 37
    factors affecting 35
    not same as tinnitus 38
Spouse, importance of 115
Stapedectomy, tinnitus with failed surgery 151
Stapedial muscle spasm 148
    tenotomy 148
Stapedius reflex 22
Stapes mobilization 150
Steroids 176
    injections into ear 179
Stimulated otoacoustic emissions from the
    cochlea 22, 34
Stress 113
    management 170
Stria vascularis 145
Stroke, fear of 114
Stubborn beliefs 157
Stump neuroma 98
Subclinical tinnitus 134
Substances applied to the ear 5
Sudden onset tinnitus 60
Suffering 159
Summating potential 27
Supporting cells 96
Surgery for deafness 149
Surgery, place in tinnitus
    management 144–155
Synthesiser 78
Syphilis 6, 7, 59, 108, 186
Systemic disease, effect on tinnitus 108

Tapotement 15
Tea 180
Tegretol® 182
Telephone follow-up 47
Temporary threshold shift 34, 106
    and residual inhibition 84
Temporo-mandibular joint 22, 144, 149
Tenseness 170
Tensor tympani 149
Tests as predictors of therapeutic masking
    effect 105
Therapist 113
Therapeutic masking trials 84
Therapeutic approach depends on patients'
    needs 164
Thyroid function 108, 186
Tinnitus—
    assessment 71–95
    associated with hearing disorder 53
    characteristics in total deafness 121

in children
  continuous 132
  diagnosis 135
  dizziness 135
  symptoms 135
clinical organization 103
complaint behaviour 158
confusion with hearing aid distortion 133
and drug therapy 176–190
experience of 3000 cases 74
generation, theory of 20–45
historical aspects 1–19
intensity and psychological techniques 172
masking therapy 96–117
more troublesome in USA 49
most troublesome 103, 136
surgical management 144–155
therapist 103
troublesome 186
worse in noise 104
Tobacco 180
Tocainide® 178
  toxicity 183
'Tonal' tinnitus not a pure tone 77
Tonic water 180
Total residual inhibition 83, 105
Toxicity of drugs used in tinnitus 179
Toynbee, fatal experiment on tinnitus 18
Tranquillizers 184
Transverse sinus 146
Travelling wave 23, 24
Trepanning the mastoid 5, 7
Tricyclic antidepressant 74
  potentiate anticonvulsant 183
True tinnitus 10

Tumours, fear of 113
Tuning curves 29
Two alternative forced choice 76
Two-tone suppression 30, 36
Tympanic membrane movement 147, 148
Tympano-sympathectomy 149
Tympanotomy 151

Unsteadiness 164
Untangling the web 158

Valsalva's manoeuvre 4
Vascular pulsation, cause 7
  loops in the IAM 147
Vasodilators 179
Venous hums 138, 145
  and raised intracranial pressure 146
Vertigo and tinnitus 147
Vestibular nerve section 144, 151, 152,
  for tinnitus alone 152
Vitamins 176
  A 179
  B 108, 179

Waking tinnitus 104
  increase of tinnitus on 98
Wax 74
Weight loss 147
Whispering tinnitus 2
White noise, in masking 99
Withdrawal of drugs 186
Worry 165

Zinc deficiency 108
Zinc therapy 179